AR~~~~~~

and

RHEUMATISM

ARTHRITIS
and
RHEUMATISM

WHAT THEY ARE —
WHAT YOU CAN DO TO HELP YOURSELF

by

D. WAINWRIGHT, M.B., M.Ch.Orth., F.R.C.S., D.Sc.(Hon.)

PAPERFRONTS
ELLIOT RIGHT WAY BOOKS,
KINGSWOOD, SURREY, U.K.

Made and printed in Great Britain by Cox & Wyman, Reading

CONTENTS

ILLUSTRATIONS

PREFACE

There is a growing interest (among the general public) in understanding the diseases which affect us all from time to time. Both radio and television have large audiences for programmes dealing with medicine and public health, and children now leave school with a fairly detailed knowledge of how the body works and how it can go wrong. In such a common condition as arthritis there seemed to be a place for a book somewhere between those written for nurses and other hospital workers and the chatty booklets which deal very simply with individual rheumatic conditions. This book is an attempt to provide a more detailed understanding of the many sides of this very common problem.

As an orthopaedic surgeon I have tried to put the surgical treatment of arthritic joints in proper perspective and have all along emphasised that the right way to tackle what may be a long and protracted disease is by team work - the patient, the family doctor, the rheumatologist and the orthopaedic surgeon.

I am indebted to my old colleague Dr. T. Hothersall, Consultant Rheumatologist to the North Staffordshire Hospital Centre, for inviting me to look at many of his problem cases and with whom I shared a joint consultative clinic in rheumatic disorders for many years.

I am also grateful to my Secretary Mrs. S. Gilman for her patience and untiring efforts in deciphering and typing an almost illegible script.

D.W.

1

INTRODUCTION

SOME MEDICAL TERMS EXPLAINED

"It's only a touch of rheumatism." "It's arthritis." These are two expressions we hear so frequently to describe the aches and pains and stiffness of muscles and joints from which most people suffer at intervals during their life. For a few, however, they may be the early signs of a more serious illness.

It is important to distinguish these widely differing disorders and to make sure that you understand what the doctors are talking about.

TERMINOLOGY

Any disease which ends in -itis is an inflammation and arthron is the Greek word for a joint. Hence arthritis literally means an inflamed joint. Long before we knew anything about bacteria and viruses, the physicians of the 17th century thought that "noxious vapours" were responsible for the spread of diseases from one joint to another. Thus the word rheumatism, derived from the Greek root rheum meaning to flow, was introduced.

Rheumatism - this is the term used in everyday conversation to describe the aches and pains we experience not only in joints but in other parts of our body - the bones, muscles and associated nerves - which we call the musculo-skeletal system.

If the symptoms are confined to the joints it is called *arthritis*. There are several distinct types and some of their names sound more frightening than they really are.

(1) *Osteo-arthritis* - a slowly progressive degeneration of one or two of the larger joints of your body, e.g. the hip and knee joints. It occurs commonly in older people, and resembles the normal "wear and tear" which occurs with

increasing age. The suffix -*itis* indicates an inflammatory condition, but because there is rarely any evidence of inflammation in the joints this condition is often called *osteoarthrosis*.

(2) *Rheumatoid arthritis* - an acute inflammation of many joints, often affecting younger people and which occasionally gives rise to crippling deformities. It is quite common - the rough estimate is that there are some 150,000 sufferers in the U.K., but of those only some 15% have significant disability. *Arthritis in children* - when rheumatoid arthritis affects children it is called *Still's disease* after Dr. Still, who first described the special features of the condition, which is uncommon.

(3) *Ankylosing spondylitis* - occasionally the inflammatory changes may be confined largely to your spine and the joints between spine and pelvis, giving rise to increasing rigidity, and the disease is sometimes known as "poker back". But this is quite rare.

(4) *Infective arthritis*

(a) *Arthralgia*. Many infectious diseases are accompanied be fleeting pains in joints and muscles. Influenza and German measles (rubella) are two examples of infections with viruses which are frequently accompanied by aching in the joints. We call such aches - arthralgia, and they happen frequently.

(b) *Synovitis*. More serious infections such as typhoid fever, undulant fever and urethritis are sometimes associated with a painful swelling of the joints due to fluid collecting in the joints - the condition known as synovitis. This is a rare complication. Fluid in a joint is usually the result of an injury or strain.

(c) *Septic arthritis*. Occasionally bacteria invade the body either through the intestine, the lungs or a septic cut or abrasion, and circulate and multiply in the blood stream. They may settle down in a joint which swells rapidly and becomes tender, red and painful. This is a serious condition which if left untreated may destroy the joint and threaten life. The tense collection of fluid must be drawn off with a needle and syringe - this procedure is known as an aspiration. The contents of the syringe are examined by a bacteriologist and when the germ has been identified the patient is treated with the appropriate antibiotic.

(d)   *Tuberculous arthritis*. Until the 1940s Tuberculosis was a very common condition throughout the world. The introduction of B.C.G. vaccination and the tuberculin testing of cattle together with the use of anti-tuberculous drugs has greatly reduced the incidence of the disease in Europe and North America but it is still a serious scourge in the Developing World. When the disease spreads to the joints it results in a slow but steady destruction of the joint surface. The joint becomes swollen but unlike a septic arthritis there is little or no evidence of inflammation and because the abscess which may form around the joint is not red or warm it is called a "cold abscess". Tuberculous infection may involve the spine, giving rise to pain and stiffness of the back. Chronic swelling of a joint or persistent backache in the immigrant population in Britain may well be due to tuberculosis. It is important that the condition is diagnosed at an early stage, when it will readily respond to treatment with the appropriate antibiotic drugs.

(5)   *Gout* - this was the first rheumatic condition to be described and studied and it occurs quite frequently. The special features of gouty arthritis are that we know the cause of it and there are specific remedies to relieve the severe pain and swelling of the affected joints and keep the inflammation under control.

The sudden onset of acute pain and redness of a joint which is characteristic of the condition is due to the accumulation of excess uric acid in the body which becomes deposited as crystals in the affected joint. The big toe is the joint most commonly affected.

(6)   *Collagen diseases* - these are a group of rare diseases which are akin to rheumatoid arthritis and are also examples of auto-immune diseases (See page 46). In addition to swelling and inflammation of the joints, other body connective tissues are involved in the diseases.

(a)   *Lupus Erythematosis*. Here arthritis is associated with patches of redness and inflamation of the skin.

(b)   *Dermatomyositis*. A similar disease in which, in addition to the joints and the skin, the muscles are also involved.

(c) *Polyarteritis*. In which the small blood vessels are also affected.

THE JOINTS

The point of junction between two bones is called a joint.

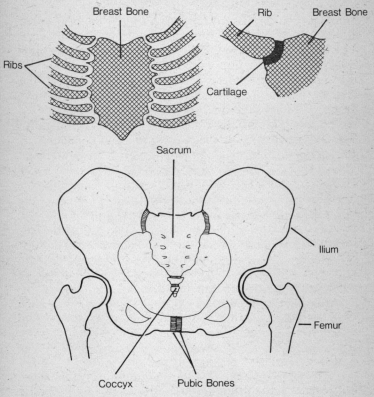

Fig. 1. Synostoses
Above: Synostoses in the front of the ribs where the breast bone is joined to the ribs.
Below: The synostoses in the pelvis between the sacrum and ilium, the sacrum and coccyx and the pubic bones. These consist of cartilage with no synovial cavity.

There are two main types - (1) *Synostosis*, (2) *Synovial joint*.

SYNOSTOSIS

Some joints like those between the bones of the skull which dovetail into each other are virtually immovable. In others, the bones are joined by firm elastic tissue we call cartilage and which can be felt in the ear flap or the tip of the nose, or by fibrous tissue. Such joints occur between the front of the ribs and the breast bone, where a small range of movement is necessary during breathing, and also at the pubis where the two halves of the pelvic bones meet in front and are joined by fibrous tissue. During pregnancy this fibrous tissue softens to allow the pelvis to expand during delivery. They have only a very limited range of movement but they can become stiff and painful in rheumatic diseases. These two examples are shown in Fig. 1.

SYNOVIAL JOINTS

Most body movement takes place at *synovial joints*. Here the bones are separated by a space lined by a thin membrane. We call this *synovial membrane* and it contains a small quantity of fluid - synovial fluid. These are the joints usually involved in arthritis. They have a remarkable structure which permits a wide range of almost frictionless movement and which normally stands up to continued use for many years. Not only do they allow movement but they provide stability. This is achieved partly by the shape of the bone ends and the way they fit together but also by the joint capsule and ligaments which join the bones together and which consist of a special type of strong fibrous tissue.

The bone ends are covered by a white shiny tissue of firm rubbery consistency which is known as *hyaline* or *articular cartilage*. It has a fine sponge-like surface through which the synovial fluid, which lubricates the joint, is pumped in and out during alternate periods of rest and activity of the joint. This fluid is contained within the delicate membrane which extends from one bone to the other and the whole is surrounded by a strong fibrous capsule which is strengthened in places by fibrous bands called ligaments. Fig. 2 illustrates how all this fits together in a knee joint.

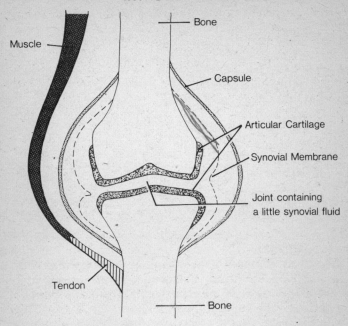

**Fig. 2. The knee joint
A typical synovial joint.**

The joint cartilage contains no nerves and is itself insensitive. However, the underlying bone and the coverings of the joint, the synovial membrane and the capsule have a rich nerve and blood supply. These are the site of the pain which is experienced in joint injuries and rheumatic diseases.

Movement of joints

The health and nutrition of your joints depend on the preservation of a normal range of movement. This helps to pump the synovial fluid in and out of the joint and avoids pressure on a particular area of cartilage. This movement is controlled by contraction and relaxation of muscles which span the joint from one bone to the next. A joint becomes painful either because the tissues lining the joint are inflamed or because the cartilage covering the bone ends is worn away.

In an attempt to protect the painful joint from movement the muscles subconsciously tighten or, as doctors say, go into spasm. The affected joint is then held in a position of relaxation where there is least tension on the inflamed tissues. In the case of the knee this is about 20° of flexion so that anyone with an arthritic knee will walk with the joint slightly bent. The constant contraction of the muscles controlling movement of a joint considerably increases the pressure within the joint which occurs whenever weight is taken through the joint. As the muscle contractions become less frequent the muscles weaken and waste. Much of the prolonged treatment required in rheumatic joints is designed to strengthen the wasted muscles.

The human joint is indeed a remarkable piece of engineering. It has a unique system of lubrication and unless injured or diseased is designed to continue moving through a wide range of movement for very many years. It has been estimated that because of the contraction of powerful muscles which control movement the human hip joint is designed to withstand pressures equivalent to over five times the body weight!

NON-ARTICULAR RHEUMATISM

Rheumatology is the name now given to the medical speciality concerned with your care if you suffer from a whole range of disorders affecting the joints and their associated structures, the muscles, tendons and the connective tissue which lies between the various specialised organs.

All of these are responsible for aches and pains of varying intensity and duration and are included in the general term rheumatism. It is true that the most important group of the rheumatic diseases involves the joints, but the word "rheumatism" embraces a large number of disorders in which the joints are unaffected and which we call soft-tissue or *non-articular rheumatism.*

Although these conditions are not serious and often clear up in a few days they are common and responsible for much minor incapacity and time off work. So, apart from joints, other parts of the body may be affected by attacks of pain, swelling and tenderness which we call rheumatism and which have specific names depending on the areas affected.

(1) Fibrositis

Beneath the skin and distributed throughout your body is a simplified form of tissue which holds together the more specialised parts of the body. This is called *connective tissue* or *fibrous tissue*. In certain areas of your body, notably under the foot, there is a concentration or thickening of this supportive tissue into stronger bands and sheets. These help to strengthen the framework of your body and in particular to contain the muscles when contracting.

This modified form of fibrous tissue is known as *fascia* and in certain parts of your body (in particular your heel, neck and the lower part of your back) may be the site of localised painful areas which we call *fibrositis* or *fasciitis*, and this occurs quite commonly.

(2) Tenosynovitis

So that muscles may perform their function of moving a joint when they contract in response to a nerve impulse, they have to have a firm attachment to the bone. The soft fleshy muscle fibres end in a smooth strong white fibrous tissue called a *tendon* which is firmly attached to the fibrous covering of the bone known as the *periosteum*. Many of these tendons move in sheaths in the shape of a tunnel. When you use muscle and tendon frequently for long periods, the tendon or more frequently the tendon sheath may become swollen and painful. For example unaccustomed prolonged use of shears to cut a hedge or any occupation which involves repeated rotation movements of the wrist and forearm may cause swelling and discomfort in the tendons over the back of the wrist. Similar symptoms may occur as a result of an inflammation of the tendon sheath. This condition is called *tendonitis* or *tenosynovitis*, a common condition.

(3) Polymalgia Rheumatica

This is the name given to an uncommon condition usually seen in older patients, chiefly women. They complain of pain and stiffness more severe in the morning which affects the muscles around the shoulder girdle and the upper arms and also the buttocks and thighs. It is an inflammatory condition affecting the muscles. The joints themselves are not involved.

It is sometimes associated with an inflammatory condition of the arteries, particularly around the temple, in which case patients also complain of severe headaches. The disease responds dramatically to treatment with cortisone (See page 52).

(4) Bursitis

A *bursa* is a small sac of thin membrane which contains fluid resembling synovial fluid. Its purpose is to protect a tendon or ligament from being damaged by friction of

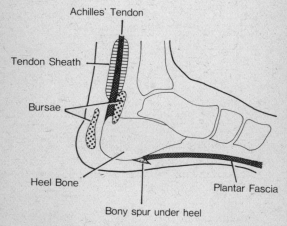

Achilles' Tendon

Tendon Sheath

Bursae

Heel Bone

Plantar Fascia

Bony spur under heel

Fig. 3.   Non-articular rheumatism
The various tissues which may be affected are illustrated in this picture of the lower part of the leg, the ankle joint and the foot.

another tendon or by underlying bone. As a result of long continued pressure or friction, or the inflammation of rheumatoid arthritis, the fluid contents increase and the bursa enlarges to form a swelling which can be seen as a bump and felt beneath the skin. We call this common condition bursitis and Fig. 3 shows a bursa lying between the heel tendon and

the heel bone and an enlarged bursa between the heel bone
and the overlying skin.

Another example of this type of bursa is the soft fluctuant
swelling which is sometimes seen in front of the knee-cap in

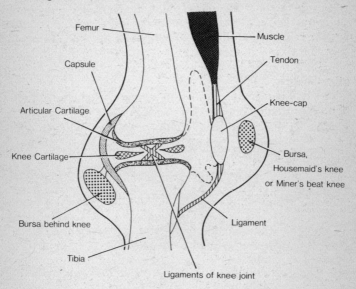

Fig. 4.   Bursitis of the knee
This can take the form of "housemaid's knee" or of a
bursa behind the joint.

those whose occupation involves a lot of kneeling. In days
gone by this used to be called "housemaid's knee" or, in the
case of coal miners, "beat knee".

A *bunion* is a bursa which develops over the prominent bone
which forms the inner side of a deformed big toe joint. Its
purpose is to protect the bone from pressure of the shoe but
the bursa itself may become inflamed from too much
pressure.

Another type of bursa sometimes occurs when the synovial
membrane of a swollen arthritic joint protrudes through the
capsule of the joint under pressure from the excess synovial

fluid. A swelling forms beneath the skin which contains synovial fluid and which communicates with the joint. Fig. 4 illustrates this type of bursa in a common site behind the knee.

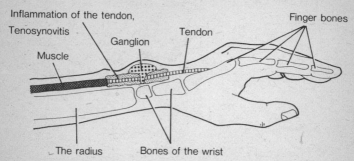

Fig. 5   The wrist
This picture illustrates a ganglion and tenosynovitis.

Perhaps the commonest example of this type of swelling is known as a *ganglion*. It is frequently seen as a firm fluctuant swelling over the back of the wrist as in Fig. 5, and arises either from the joints between the small bones of the wrist or from the tendon sheaths.

(5)   Capsulitis

As we have seen, a synovial joint consists of two adjacent bone ends, each covered by firm smooth cartilage, joined by the delicate synovial membrane (which normally extrudes a small amount of viscid fluid for lubrication) and by strong ligaments.

The whole joint is protected by a covering of thickened fibrous tissue which we call *the capsule*. When a joint is injured, strained or used excessively for a long period the joint lining reacts by producing an excess of synovial fluid. This is called a *synovitis* and is accompanied by swelling and pain and stiffness of the joint. Similar changes may occur as a result of inflammation of the synovial membrane due to some infection or injury.

As the fluid in the affected joint is gradually absorbed, the folds of the synovial membrane and the capsule of the joint

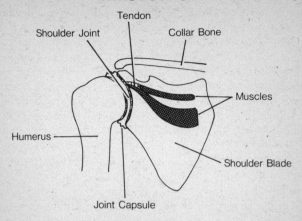

Tendon

Shoulder Joint

Collar Bone

Muscles

Humerus

Shoulder Blade

Joint Capsule

Fig. 6. The shoulder joint
When this is affected by inflammation it produces an
excess of synovial fluid and adhesions are formed
limiting the range of movement, a condition called
capsulitis or frozen shoulder.

form *adhesions* limiting the range of movement. We call this
condition "*capsulitis*" and it is particularly liable to affect the
shoulder joint shown in Fig. 6 which becomes very stiff and
painful This common condition is often referred to as a
"frozen shoulder".

(6) Tennis elbow
   This is explained fully on page 100.

(7) Neuritis
   The nerves of your body have two important functions.
They conduct the stimuli which arise in your brain or spinal
cord to activate the muscles, and they convey sensation (e.g.
touch, pain and sense of position) from your skin and
subcutaneous tissues to the brain.
   Stimulation of a nerve by undue pressure or inflammation
arising from some general infection gives rise to pain over the
particular area of the body which the nerve supplies. The pain
is often severe of a sharp stabbing nature and aggravated by

movement or pressure. It is called *neuritis* or sometimes *neuralgia,* and happens quite frequently.

(a)   *Brachial neuritis and Sciatica*

The nerve roots which arise from your spinal cord in the region of your neck or the lower part of your back are particularly vulnerable to pressure or irritation as they emerge through small holes between the vertebrae close to the joints between the vertebrae. If these joints are rough and irregular as a result of arthritis these holes will be narrowed and in addition to pain in your neck or back, you will experience radiating pain down your arm or leg. These two

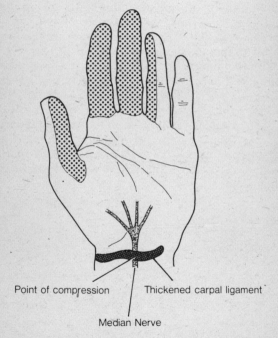

Point of compression   Thickened carpal ligament

Median Nerve

Fig. 7. The hand and wrist
This picture illustrates carpal tunnel syndrome where the median nerve is compressed by a thickened carpal ligament. The shaded area is the part of the hand affected by tingling and numbness.

common painful disorders are called *brachial neuritis* in the arm and *sciatica* in the leg.

(b) *Carpal Tunnel Syndrome*

Another common type of neuritis is caused by pressure on the median nerve, one of the main nerves running down your arm and in front of your wrist to supply the small muscles in your hand and provide sensation to the outer part of your hand and fingers. This nerve is closely related to the tendons which run down in front of your wrist to move your fingers. In rheumatoid arthritis and certain other generalised diseases these tendon sheaths become thickened and swollen, trapping the nerve between the tendons and ligament. This gives rise to tingling and numbness of your thumb, index, middle and part of your "ring" finger as illustrated in Fig. 7, and wasting of the small muscles in your hand with consequent weakness of grip. This condition is known as the *carpal tunnel syndrome*, and is quite common.

The pain is often worse at night or when your arm is hanging down. It is relieved by applying a light splint to your wrist at night and may be improved by injecting hydrocortisone into the tissues around the nerve at your wrist.

If, however, the pain persists, complete relief can be obtained by releasing the nerve from pressure by dividing the thickened ligament lying in front of the nerve at the wrist - a small operation with a quick recovery.

2

METHODS OF TREATMENT

Intractable pain sometimes accompanied by swelling are probably the symptoms for which you consult your doctor. It is important that you describe these symptoms as clearly as possible. Where is the pain? Where does it radiate? What type of pain is it? - a dull continuous ache, an intermittent sharp pain or a tingling sensation.

What brings on the pain and what makes it worse, e.g. a particular movement?

Is it worse at night or is it relieved by lying down?

These are the sort of questions the doctor will ask as he takes a careful history. He will examine the painful area and other joints, followed by a general physical examination to exclude any general disease which may be responsible for the symptoms, e.g. infectious diseases, heart or kidney disease, influenza or even a sore throat.

Once the diagnosis has been established treatment will consist of local measures and the use of drugs which relieve pain – analgesic drugs.

Analgesic drugs

Only the milder group of drugs is required for the relief of pain in muscular rheumatism. Aspirin is the most readily available and most effective drug for minor pain, provided the patient does not suffer from a gastric disorder, asthma or any tendency to bleed easily. It should be taken in doses of two 0.3 gram tablets every four to six hours for a maximum of ten days. Remember aspirin can irritate the stomach and should not be taken by anyone suffering from a peptic ulcer. It can also interfere with the normal clotting of blood and should not be used by anyone who has a tendency to excessive bleeding.

Two other mild analgesics in common use are Paracetamol (Panadol) and Distalgesic tablets – both of which are usually well tolerated and can be taken safely for short periods.

LOCAL TREATMENT

1. *Rest and splinting*

When the condition is acute you have got to rest the painful area and keep it elevated and avoid weight-bearing until the

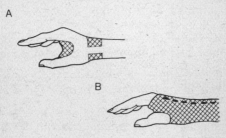

Fig. 8.   Splints
For (A) thumb and (B) wrist. These are used to rest painful joints while the inflammation is acute. Usually made of aluminium, plaster of Paris or light-weight plastic material.

pain settles down. If the joint is very painful your doctor may advise supporting the limb in a sling or light splint. Some examples of splints are shown in Fig. 8. They are usually made of light malleable metal, e.g. aluminium padded for comfort or plaster of Paris moulded to the limb above and below the joint. There are, however, a number of light-weight plastic materials which can be moulded to a painful joint after heating or immersing in hot water and when cooled have the added advantage of being lighter than plaster and impervious to water.

In addition to resting a painful joint, splints may be used to correct a deformity, e.g. a bent arthritic knee joint may be rested in plaster and after a few days the plaster is removed, the joint gradually straightened by a gentle manipulation and a new plaster applied in the maximum degree of correction, as shown in Fig. 9.

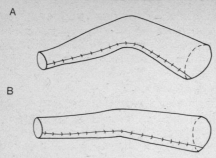

Fig. 9.   Leg splints
A bent arthritic knee may be rested in plaster such as A. After a few days the plaster is removed, the joint is gradually straightened by gentle manipulation and a new plaster (B) is applied in the maximum degree of correction.

To prevent permanent stiffness the period during which a painful arthritic joint is rested completely should only be sufficient for the acute pain and swelling to settle down – often no more than a few days. The splint should then be removed at intervals at first under the guidance of a physiotherapist to practise assisted active movements which will later be carried out at home.

2.   *Physiotherapy*
When the acute phase has subsided a skilled experienced physiotherapist may use physical aids and movements to improve function. This is a very important factor in the treatment of any disorder.

Painful rheumatic conditions are accompanied by protective spasm of muscles followed by joint stiffness, and the aim of the various types of physiotherapy is to relieve muscle spasm and gradually restore a painless range of movement.

(a)   *Heat and cold*
When the joint is hot and tender, ice-packs will help to reduce the inflammation, but when the acute stage is subsiding heat applied in the form of hot moist packs or a

covered hot water bottle will improve the deep circulation and diminish muscle spasm. Other more sophisticated ways of heating up the deeper tissues are the use of an infra-red lamp or short-wave diathermy and ultrasound.

(b) *Infra-red treatment*

Infra-red rays are that portion of the light spectrum which produces radiant heat. They merely heat the superficial tissues of the body and possess no mysterious or unusual properties. Although a number of special infra-red generators are marketed, an ordinary electrical household heater makes a fair substitute for an infra-red lamp except that the latter has a coned reflector which concentrates the heat on a particular area.

(c) *Short-wave diathermy*

When alternating electric current of moderately high frequency is applied to the body it produces an electric shock and a severe contraction of the muscles. However, if the frequency is increased to over 10,000 oscillations per second (by special apparatus in a hospital) the muscles cease to contract and no shock is experienced. On the other hand local heat is generated because the body tissues offer varying degrees of resistance to the flow of the current and such heat can penetrate the deeper tissues to a distance of 6 cms.

(d) *Ultrasonic therapy*

More recently apparatus has been devised to apply very high frequency sound waves to small localised areas of the body. These have an effect on connective tissue by producing local heat and breaking up more rigid types of fibrous tissue. This type of treatment is particularly effective when dealing with adhesions around a joint, e.g. tennis elbow.

(e) *Exercises*

The exercises are graded according to the stage of the condition. In the early phase "passive" movements are done by the physiotherapist while you are relaxed. As the condition becomes less painful you are encouraged to move the joints with some assistance. Finally you perform full free active exercises against resistance.

All physiotherapy departments are overcrowded and physiotherapists are in short supply, so the aim of treatment must be to teach you to perform the exercises regularly at home with the assistance of relatives.

Some of these exercises are illustrated in other chapters, see pages 61 to 63.

(f) *Manipulation*

When the acute painful stage of muscle or joint inflammation has settled down, you may find that chronic stiffness of a joint persists. This may be due to adhesions forming between the delicate joint lining and the surrounding tissues, or a shortening and loss of elasticity of the ligaments or muscles controlling movement. If these do not respond to treatment by heat and graduated exercises, it may be necessary for the physiotherapist or the doctor to use a degree of controlled force to move the joint. This is known as a manipulation and may be performed under anaesthesia or more commonly without an anaesthetic.

In addition to stretching or breaking down joint adhesions, manipulation is also used to correct minor degrees of joint displacement which may be associated with injury or degeneration or cartilage tissue lying between two bones. For example, it may be appropriate for torn and displaced cartilages in the knee joint, or the cartilage discs which join the vertebral bones of the spine and which, particularly in the neck or lumbar spine, may cause pressure on the nerves as they emerge from the spinal cord.

This treatment should only be undertaken by physiotherapists or doctors specially trained in this technique and only after a full clinical examination and X-rays have excluded the possibility of a more serious underlying disease as the cause of the persistent pain or disability. This applies particularly to the spine. Here, injudicious and over-vigorous manipulation in the wrong sort of case may result in increasing the pressure on nerve roots or even the spinal cord, with the possibility of permanent weakness of the legs or even paralysis.

(g) *Traction*

This is another form of physical treatment which is becoming increasingly popular. It is an attempt to relieve pain by distracting (pulling apart) two adjacent bones and is often used as a preliminary manoeuvre before manipulating a joint. It is applied to the spine in an attempt to relieve the pressure on the nerve roots which may be caused by arthritic changes in the spinal joints or torn or displaced intervertebral discs. Brachial neuritis or sciatica are the two conditions for which traction is particularly useful.

Intermittent traction is performed in the physiotherapy department using a halter with traction straps attached to a weight over a pulley at the end of the couch for neck and arm pain or a corset around the pelvis in the case of low back pain with sciatica. In more severe cases it is better to use continuous traction for two or three weeks but this requires admission to a hospital bed.

A useful method of finding out whether traction is likely to benefit low back pain and sciatica is for you to grasp the top of an open door and swing loosely with your feet off the ground for a few minutes. The weight of the body will act as a downward force on the lumbar spine and frequently results in temporary relief of the pain.

(h) *Electrical treatment*

All painful conditions prevent normal contraction of muscles which soon become weak and wasted. The rapid wasting seen in the thigh muscles accompanying a painful swollen knee is a good example. This muscle weakness will gradually improve if you learn actively to contract the muscles controlling the joint movement. When difficulty is experienced in initiating movement, it is helpful if the physiotherapist stimulates the affected muscle with faradic (interrupted) current. Such contractions help to maintain the strength and tone of the muscles until you can perform active contractions yourself.

3. *Acupuncture*

This is a traditional form of treatment introduced by the

Chinese to the Western world and is now in popular use for the treatment of local and referred pain. Although its scientific basis has not been established there seems no doubt that in some people suffering from soft-tissue disorders, particularly backache, rapid relief of pain may follow the introduction of fine needles to certain acupuncture points in the body. It is possible that the explanation for the relief of pain may be similar to the use of a counter-irritant where the stimulation of superficial nerve endings may inhibit the pain in deeper nerve fibres.

We do not fully understand the mechanism of feeling pain. Under great stress, such as wartime conditions, pain associated with severe injuries is not always experienced, and intense pain can often be diminished by psychotherapy and hypnosis. Stimulation of one set of nerves either by acupuncture or electrical impulses applied to the skin may temporarily prevent other painful stimuli from being conducted to the brain. This is known as the gate-control theory.

Over the centuries the Chinese have built up a map or pattern of "acupuncture points" and fine gold or silver needles are inserted into the skin and sometimes deeper until they touch bone - the site varying according to the type of pain experienced.

The relief experienced is often temporary and does not work for some people but it has the great advantage that it is harmless when done properly *under full aseptic conditions*, which is more than can be said for many other forms of treatment both orthodox and unorthodox.

4.   *Aspiration of synovial fluid*

All joints lined by synovial membrane react to injury, infection or rheumatic disease by a rapid increase in the amount of synovial fluid in the joint leading to a large swelling which may become tense and painful.

Small effusions will subside with rest but large collections of fluid may require the insertion of a hollow needle under local anaesthesia through which the excess fluid can be drawn into a syringe. This procedure is known as aspiration of a joint and is a necessary preliminary to injecting the joint with an anti-inflammatory drug.

5. *Injection treatment*

Small localised tender nodules which are often seen in muscular rheumatism may respond to injections of local anaesthesia alone. However, local injection of one of the corticosteroid drugs is now used, either alone or in combination with a local anaesthetic, for the relief of rheumatic pain arising around a joint or from the joint itself.

Corticosteroids provide the most rapid method of relieving inflammation in joints or the ligaments and capsule such as tenosynovitis or "tennis elbow". The usual preparation used for local injection is hydrocortisone and, provided full aseptic precautions are taken, the injection of small doses occasionally into or around painful joints which are not responding to the usual remedies often produces a dramatic relief of symptoms. The swelling subsides, the redness and tenderness disappears and the function of the joint improves. Care must be exercised in repeating these injections in weight-bearing joints, e.g. the knee joint, as the articular cartilage may later undergo increasing wear. With these precautions in mind local injection of steroid preparations has proved to be one of the most significant advances in the treatment of rheumatic conditions.

3

BACKACHE AND ARTHRITIS OF THE SPINE

It is not surprising that the back is the source of more pain and disability than any other part of the body. The spinal column consists of 24 mobile vertebrae, each joined to the other by three joints, and all may be the site of arthritis (such as in Fig. 11 A), degenerative changes or injury. Running through a triangular tunnel formed by the body of the vertebrae in front and the laminae behind is the spinal cord from which the spinal nerves emerge on either side of each bony vertebra.

The main nerves which serve the arm (brachial) and leg (sciatic) are shown in Fig. 10.

Your spine has to be strong yet supple and it is subjected to constant abnormal stresses and strains particularly if you are engaged in heavy manual work. Because it forms a major part of the skeleton it is often involved to some degree in any generalised illness which affects bones and joints.

"*Lumbago*" really means lumbar backache and is the term used to describe the common low back pain produced by undue fatigue or strain and bad postures at work.

These postural aches usually respond to rest on a firm mattress, local heat and mild analgesic tablets. If they recur frequently they are probably associated with some abnormal wear and tear in the ligaments or joints of the spine or the intervertebral discs.

"SLIPPED" DISC

One of the commonest causes of recurrent attacks of low back pain is a tear or displacement of the cartilage pad which joins together the main part of the bones - known as the

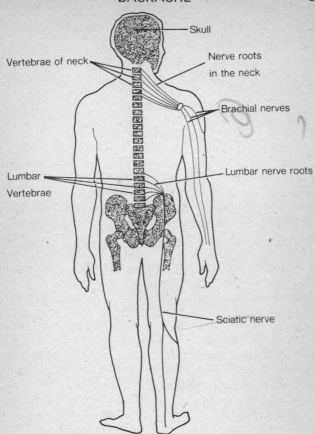

Fig. 10. The spine
The vertebrae of the spine, and how the nerves issue from them to serve the arms and legs.

vertebral body. These flat circular pads of cartilage are known as intervertebral discs - or simply discs - and consist of an outer casing of gristle surrounding a jelly-like substance and are sufficiently flexible to allow movement in all directions and also to act as shock-absorbers. The lower part of the back is particularly liable to excessive strains and here in the lumbar

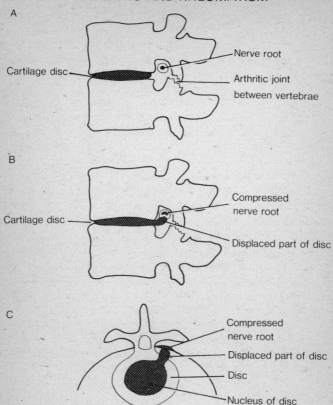

Fig. 11.   The vertebrae

      A   Side view of two normal vertebrae showing the cartilage disc but with an arthritic joint between the vertebrae.

      B   Side view of two lumbar vertebrae showing a displaced (slipped) disc and how it compresses the nerve root.

      C   How this looks from above.

region the discs are thicker and stronger. In older people they become thinner and lose some of their elasticity.

When you stoop forward suddenly to lift a heavy weight,

particularly if the knees are kept straight, the discs in the lumbar region are subjected to a severe strain and the outer casing of the disc may give way allowing the central portion to displace backwards where it can slip to one side and press on one of the nerves as it emerges from the spinal canal, as shown in Figs. 11 B and C.

Rupture of the disc causes sudden severe pain in the back and if the nerve root is compressed severe pain is also experienced in parts served by the affected nerve.

By far the commonest discs to be involved are the two lower discs in the lumbar region, and irritation of the nerve roots here causes pain referred down the leg, usually the back of the thigh and outer part of the calf. As these nerve roots join together to form the sciatic nerve, pain with this type of distribution is known as sciatica. The pain may be very severe. The back may be stiff. The ability to raise the leg from the horizontal position may be limited and there is occasionally numbness of the lower part of the leg and foot.

Although the disc is usually damaged by a violent strain of the back when lifting heavy objects it may occur in older people who normally lead sedentary lives and suddenly take up heavy tasks such as gardening. The disc may be damaged by repeated minor strains and the final tear occurs during a quite trivial action, such as getting out of bed or stooping over a wash basin.

TREATMENT

In the acute phase bed rest is essential. This should be as complete as possible on a firm mattress, using a board under it if necessary, and should continue for several weeks until the pain subsides. This relaxes the back muscles which are in painful spasm and protects the torn disc tissue from further damage and allows healing to occur by the formation of scar tissue.

Until the back muscles relax it is better to adopt the most comfortable position, usually lying on the side with the knees and hips bent up, but as the spasm subsides you should try to lie flat with the back supported on a firm mattress and the knees supported with a pillow as shown in Fig. 12 B. Your

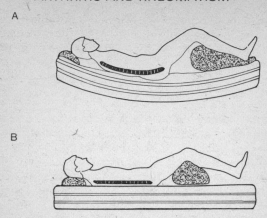

Fig. 12. Resting
   A (Above) The WRONG position.
   B (Below) The RIGHT position.

doctor will prescribe pain-relieving and sedative tablets and it is important to take these early in the attack in sufficient doses to relieve the pain and ensure a good night's rest. Most attacks will settle with treatment on these lines for a few weeks. Some aching and stiffness often persists and the back remains vulnerable to further strains. After any severe attack it is advisable to wear a light support to the back such as a canvas corset reinforced with steel strips. The object is to restrict sudden movements of the lumbar spine and protect the torn disc as it heals.

At the same time it is important to strengthen the back muscles by regularly carrying out simple exercises; the most effective is to lie flat on the back with hands behind the head and practise raising the feet with the knees straight. They should be held in this position for a few seconds and then slowly lowered. The exercise is repeated ten times and gradually increased each day until you can do it twenty times.

Correct lifting is important. The lumbar spine is held rigid by contracting the back muscles and the object to be lifted which should lie close to your feet is reached by bending the hips and knees, as in Fig. 13 B. A heavy object is then slowly lifted on to the knees and then supported by the arms in front of the chest. This is achieved without bending the back. The hips and knees are then slowly straightened to regain the upright position.

A   B

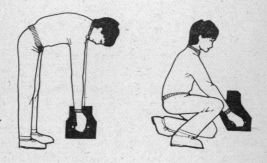

Fig. 13.   Lifting
A   The WRONG way.
B   The RIGHT way.

If the original acute attack of pain does not settle or if the symptoms continue to recur your doctor will probably refer you to hospital for further investigation and treatment.

X-RAYS

In addition to the ordinary X-rays of the spine, a myelogram may be required. This consists of X-rays of the spine taken after a special dye which is opaque to X-rays has been injected into the sheath which covers the spinal cord. The flow of this fluid up and down the spine can be seen on a viewing screen and any disturbance of normal flow will indicate the site and size of a disc protrusion.

INJECTIONS

Most cases of low back pain, with or without sciatic

radiation, settle down with adequate rest, support and limiting activities for some time. Acute attacks which do not subside with simple conservative measures may respond to the injection of a local anaesthetic into the tissues around the spinal nerve roots – these are known as epidural injections.

TRACTION

Traction to the spine by means of a broad band applied to the pelvis to which weights can be attached not only ensures complete rest but overcomes spasm of the spinal muscles and may increase the space between the vertebral bones and restore the displaced disc to its normal position. Continuous traction can only be applied in hospital but as an out-patient periods of intermittent traction can be applied by physio-therapists, and this often proves helpful when recovery is slow.

SPINAL MANIPULATION

Less acute cases may respond to a rotation manipulation of the spine aimed at repositioning the displaced disc and freeing the nerve root of pressure. This manoeuvre is only indicated if there is no evidence of severe root pressure. Injudicious spinal manipulations on the wrong case may make matters worse, so manipulation should only be undertaken after a full neurological examination, and carried out by doctors or physiotherapists experienced in this type of treatment.

OPERATION

The operation involves removal of a portion of the bones and ligaments over the affected area, displacing the spinal cord to one side and removing the displaced portion of the disc. It often results in a dramatic relief of the constant pain but in a small number of cases the relief may only be temporary and complications do occur occasionally. Operative treatment is reserved for a relatively small number of people who continue to have intractable pain in spite of adequate conservative treatment.

Even after removal of the disc it is unwise to continue heavy work in which the back is subjected to continued strain.

Arthritis of the spine

There are two very different types of arthritis of the spine.

1. *Ankylosing spondylitis*

This rare condition affects young people, usually men in their twenties, and resembles rheumatoid arthritis. Like disc trouble, with which it is sometimes confused in its early stage, it starts with attacks of pain and stiffness in the back. It is

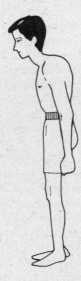

**Fig. 14. Ankylosing spondylitis
The appearance of an advanced case.**

called ankylosing spondylitis from Spondylos, the Greek word for spine and ankylos - stiffness, and, because in its advanced stage it gives rise to a very rigid spine, it is sometimes called "poker back".

Inflammatory changes similar to those seen in rheumatoid arthritis (see Chapter 4, page 43) affect the joints between the vertebrae starting in the lumbar spine and the pelvis and spreading upwards to affect the lumbar and thoracic spine and sometimes the neck. The attacks of back pain and muscle spasm are accompanied by stiffness of the spine, loss of the normal spinal curves, and patients may develop a stoop.

When recognised and treated in the early stages the disease may be limited to stiffness of the lower part of the back but in a few cases the whole spine becomes involved and occasionally the hip and shoulder joints, giving rise to considerable deformity and great difficulty in walking. Although some of the blood tests are abnormal the specific tests for rheumatoid arthritis are not present. X-rays do not show the typical destructive changes of rheumatoid arthritis but the affected joints can become fused and may join up completely.

If untreated, people with this disease are recognised by round shoulders and a bend in the back which throws considerable strain on the neck when they look up. They have increasing difficulty in turning the head and shoulders round and crossing the road or backing a car becomes hazardous, so every effort must be made to keep the spine mobile and as straight as possible.

The cause of the disease, like the majority of rheumatic conditions, is unknown and there is no specific cure, but much can be done to limit the deformity and stiffness by regular exercises and careful attention to correct posture. Very often the disease settles down in a few years, leaving perhaps little more than some stiffness of the back.

Treatment

If this condition is recognised in its early stage, with modern treatment the outlook is good and you may not even lose a day's work. Only in very few cases does severe disability arise. It is essential to keep the spine as mobile as possible and all forms of prolonged rigid fixation, e.g. a plaster jacket, should be avoided. You are taught progressive spinal exercises designed to maintain a good posture and improve the chest expansion; these must be practised regularly at home.

A firm mattress is essential and under-water exercises and swimming are particularly beneficial. The exercises are illustrated in Figs. 15 and 16. They must be performed regularly, each movement repeated twelve times and will take up to ten-fifteen minutes preferably twice a day, once after a

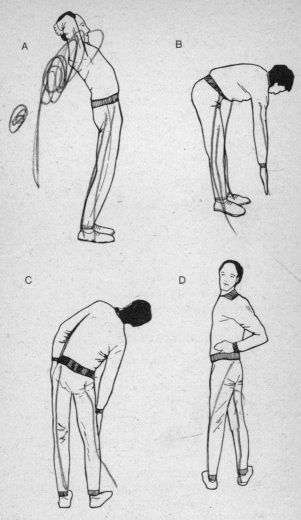

Fig. 15. Exercises for the spine
A & B   Bend backwards and forwards.
C   Bend sideways.
D   Rotate about the hips.

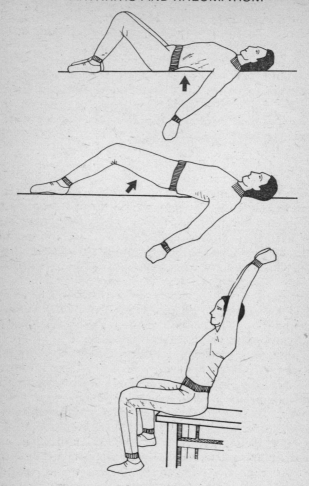

Fig. 16. More exercises for the spine
    A Lying with the knees raised, lift the small of
        the back.
    B Lift the buttocks.
    C Sitting on a bench, bend backwards and
        forwards with arms raised.

hot bath. They are designed to keep the neck, dorsal and lumbar spine as freely movable as possible and in addition full movements of the hips and knees should be practised.

You must realise that relief from the pain and stiffness lies largely with yourself and that drugs are only a means of helping you to perform the exercises more thoroughly. Both analgesic and anti-inflammatory drugs, e.g. aspirin and indomethacin, are prescribed during the acute phase and any subsequent painful attacks, but steroid drugs are never indicated.

2.   *Osteo-arthritis of the spine*

Unlike the inflammatory type of spinal arthritis discussed above, osteo-arthritis or degenerative arthritis of the spine is a common condition and most people over the age of sixty show signs of it in the back or the neck. It is more likely to occur at an earlier age if you have some deformity of the spine such as a round back, hollow back and particularly if the spine is bent sideways, a condition doctors call *scoliosis*.

X-rays show that the spaces between the vertebrae are narrowed and bony spurs are seen projecting from the edges of the bones which encroach on the gaps between adjacent bones through which the spinal nerves emerge.

In addition to progressive stiffness of the back you will, if you are a sufferer, complain of pain down the legs and into the neck, shoulders and arms. The condition is more common in men who have been engaged in heavy manual work and in sedentary workers it is aggravated by unaccustomed activity such as digging or hedge-clipping. The degenerative changes may affect the cartilage discs which cushion the spine and allow mobility, and tearing and protrusion of these discs can give rise to all the signs and symptoms of the so-called "slipped" disc which is more commonly seen in younger people following an injury.

TREATMENT

Avoid sudden bursts of strenuous exercise and adopt a correct posture when engaged in any activity likely to throw a strain on the back. Sit in chairs with the back well-supported;

lift from the knees and the hips with the back well-controlled; sleep on firm mattresses, and, when the neck is involved, use only one pillow to support the head.

Pain-relieving tablets and sleeping tablets may be required when the pain is acute but do not take these for long periods. We are dealing with a chronic disability and the dangers of habit-forming and drug addiction are very real.

Most attacks of backache clear up with simple, almost self-evident measures. Local heat, e.g. a hot water bottle and hot baths relieve muscle spasm and many patients will be helped by the temporary use of a light well-fitting corset.

4

RHEUMATOID ARTHRITIS

Arthritis is an age-old disease. There is evidence of it in the fossilised skeletons of Dinosaurs and Neolithic man, and history records that among many famous people of the past who suffered from arthritis were Julius Caesar, Frederick the Great, and Catherine di Medici.

Arthritis in its varied forms is probably the commonest of all diseases and has accounted for more prolonged disability and loss of work than any other disorder. Nevertheless it is only during the last thirty years that intensive research into the cause of the disease, and scientific evaluation of its treatment have been conducted on a large scale.

Many people have a friend or relative crippled with arthritis and whenever they get a painful swollen joint are anxious lest this is the beginning of a similar condition.

Osteo-arthritis is mainly caused by the wear and tear occurring with advancing years in joints which, in some cases, have been abnormal from childhood. By contrast *rheumatoid arthritis* is a generalised inflammatory disease which affects many organs throughout the body including the joints. It is the joint involvement which produces the characteristic signs and symptoms and which is responsible for the crippling disability which occasionally develops.

Onset and course of rheumatoid arthritis

The disease usually starts as a mild aching or stiffness, often more noticeable in the morning and accompanied by a general feeling of being "run-down" and tired. Although any age may be affected it occurs more commonly in women of middle age. During the course of the disease the joints may suddenly flare up, becoming swollen and tender, and unlike osteo-arthritis those most frequently involved are the smaller more remote joints such as the fingers and wrists or the joints of the foot. Any of the joints, however, may be involved and it is not uncommon for symptoms to settle down in the hands or fingers and re-appear in the elbow or shoulder. When pain and stiffness of joints continue to recur in this way rheumatoid arthritis must be suspected and you need a full medical investigation since treatment in the early stage of the disease, before permanent changes in the joints have occurred, is much more effective.

The inflammation of the joint mainly affects the synovium or joint lining. This becomes engorged with small dilated blood vessels and is slowly converted from a fine delicate membrane to thickened swollen tissue which can be felt to bulge around the edges of the joint and which may destroy the smooth cartilage on which the normal gliding movements of the joint take place. This is accompanied by a marked increase in the amount of fluid in the joint with stretching of the ligaments which stabilise the joint, giving rise to laxity and deformity.

Diagnosis:

Pain and swelling of several smaller joints of the body accompanied by a generalised stiffness which comes and goes over a period of several weeks is highly suggestive of rheumatoid arthritis.

Unless the condition has been present for some time X-rays of the joints may not show anything abnormal. On the other hand if the disease has been present for many months the bones become less calcified, the joint space narrowed and the joint surfaces irregular and eroded, and these changes can be detected by X-rays.

Your doctor has at his disposal other investigations which may help to establish a diagnosis:

Blood tests

The rate at which the red and white blood cells settle in a column of blood in a fine tube in a given time is increased in all active inflammatory diseases, and a raised sedimentation rate, as it is called and a degree of anaemia (a low haemoglobin) are almost always present in active rheumatoid disease.

Another blood test which is also helpful is the test which establishes the presence or absence of an abnormal protein in the blood, known as the rheumatoid factor – this is present in 80% of patients suffering from rheumatoid arthritis.

Examination of synovial fluid

The amount of synovial fluid is greatly increased in joints affected by arthritis, particularly rheumatoid arthritis, and it is often sticky and yellow in colour. It can be assessed and examined by drawing off the fluid with a fine needle and syringe under local anaesthesia.

These and other tests will help your doctor to decide whether he is dealing with a case of rheumatoid arthritis but if doubt persists a portion of the joint lining – the synovial membrane – may be removed and examined under the microscope. This can be done by a small open operation or more frequently nowadays by inserting an instrument into the affected joint and viewing the appearance of the synovial membrane by means of an illuminated tube called an arthroscope. A small section of the membrane can also be removed for examination using this instrument.

Other signs of rheumatoid arthritis

Structures other than joints which may be involved in rheumatoid disease include tendon sheaths, and the tendons, which become swollen and tender, may rupture, giving rise to "dropped fingers or thumb" when the patient is unable to straighten the fingers.

Firm nodules sometimes form under the skin, often around the elbow joint, and occasionally ulcerate. The small blood vessels may become inflamed, leading to ulceration of the skin, and nerves become compressed by pressure of swollen rheumatoid tissue below a rigid ligament. This occurs in the carpal tunnel syndrome at the wrist, giving rise to troublesome tingling of the fingers. Occasionally the rheumatoid changes may involve the eye with increasing impairment of vision.

Cause of rheumatoid arthritis

In spite of intensive medical research through the world the cause of this common disease, like the common cold, is still unknown. The onset is often related to some physical or mental stress and may occur after childbirth or during the menopause. During pregnancy, however, arthritic symptoms frequently disappear, suggesting that disturbance of hormonal balance may play a part in the progress of the disease.

Because of the slow destructive nature of the disorder, resembling in many respects tuberculous disease of joints, it was originally thought to be due to a bacterial or virus infection and a variety of germs have been found in the joints and other tissues of patients suffering from rheumatoid arthritis. Although this infective theory has not been entirely ruled out, most research workers now feel that rheumatoid arthritis is an example of an auto-immune disease.

Auto-immunity

When the system is attacked by an invader from outside such as bacteria or viruses, there is a swift reaction by the defence mechanism of the body. Specialised blood cells called lymphocytes circulating throughout the body come into contact with the antigens, as these invaders are called, and are transformed into larger cells called plasma cells. These in turn produce antibodies which combine with and immobilise the antigens. The complex thus formed is then attacked and engulfed by another specialised blood cell - the phagocyte - a type of scavenger which breaks up and digests it.

This is the way the body overcomes any infection or toxic substance which invades it – the normal protection system.

In rheumatoid arthritis, for some reason which as yet we do not understand, the lymphocytes after combining with the antigen fail to produce sufficient antibodies and attack the cells lining the joint and also the neighbouring cartilage. The synovial membrane reacts by becoming thickened and inflamed, the cartilage covering the joint surface softens and the cells are in part destroyed. These destructive changes give rise to increasing pain, stiffness and deformity, with slowly progressive disability.

A theory of the cause of rheumatoid arthritis

Invaders called antigens possibly produced by a virus infection similar to those causing measles or German measles combine with normal cells of the body called Lymphocytes

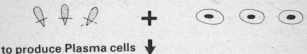

to produce Plasma cells ↓

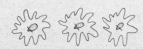

which form antibodies

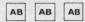

The antibodies combine with the antigens to produce a complex

which is normally destroyed by scavenging cells called Phagocytes.

In rheumatoid arthritis there is a failure to produce sufficient antibodies to combat the antigens which attack the joint lining or synovium and the underlying joint cartilage.

Fig. 17.   A theory of the cause of rheumatoid arthritis.

Arthritis may occur in several members of one family and it is now accepted that hereditary factors may have a part to play in the onset of the disease.

TREATMENT OF RHEUMATOID ARTHRITIS

There is no one form of treatment which will cure rheumatoid arthritis and successful management requires the combined skills of many people. The diagnosis and your treatment in the early stages will fall to the G.P. (General Practitioner) supported by radiological and pathological services of the nearby hospital.

If the condition does not settle down, or if the symptoms tend to recur at frequent intervals, further investigation or more specialised treatment will be required. Most hospitals now provide out-patient clinics staffed by Rheumatologists. These are physicians with considerable experience in the use of an ever-increasing range of drugs and with access to physiotherapy departments. Many of these departments organise combined clinics with Orthopaedic Surgeons where severe joint involvement and deformity can be assessed by both physicians and surgeons to see if you are likely to benefit from surgical treatment.

The type of treatment will depend on the stage of the disease when you are first seen.

In the early stage, pain and stiffness are the predominant

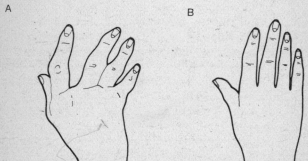

Fig. 18.   The finger joints
A   Deformity caused by rheumatoid arthritis.
B   How it can be corrected surgically.

symptoms. These may be followed later by swelling of several joints. At this stage the disease usually responds to treatment, and the swollen joints and symptoms are controlled.

Occasionally the rheumatic changes persist. If this happens instability and deformity of the joints may develop with muscle weakness and wasting. These changes are seen characteristically in your finger joints which become swollen. The fingers themselves bend sideways and the grip is weakened as shown in Fig. 18 A. Later it may be impossible to straighten your knees or raise your arms above shoulder level and gradually you can become increasingly crippled.

Although rheumatoid arthritis is a serious condition it is important to remember that *the majority of cases have little or no permanent disability.*

The degree of disability often depends on recognising the disease in its early stage, on the quality of the early treatment and on your whole-hearted co-operation in what may well be long-continued treatment and observation. It is important that you should be fully informed about the nature of the disease, and be given detailed instructions about the part you can play at home in preventing deformities and restoring movement to the affected joints.

Once the diagnosis has been established treatment will consist of measures to relieve pain and gradually reduce the degree of inflammation in the affected joints.

TREATMENT WITH DRUGS

There are two main groups of drugs which are useful.

1. *Analgesic drugs* which are purely pain-relievers.

2. *Anti-inflammatory drugs.* These are drugs which have a specific effect on those tissues affected by arthritis and help the inflammation to subside.

Because many of these drugs have to be taken for long periods and sometimes in high doses, unpleasant side-effects may develop, in particular gastric upsets, and you must always report these to the prescribing doctor.

Analgesic drugs

Panadol is one of the mildest analgesics and is usually well tolerated. It is sometimes combined with tranquillisers in the preparation known as Lobak – where the additional relaxation may benefit those suffering from painful stiff backs. Distalgesic and Codis tablets are other popular mild analgesic preparations with few side-effects.

However, most Rheumatologists believe that one of the oldest analgesic preparations, Aspirin, is the most effective drug to be prescribed in the early stages of rheumatism. Most people tolerate it well even in large doses but a few are allergic to it and it should not be prescribed if you suffer from a gastric ulcer, or asthma, or have a tendency to bleed excessively.

In small doses it acts purely as a pain reliever but in larger doses it acts also as an anti-inflammatory drug.

Anti-inflammatory drugs

There are a wide range of drugs which have a special place in the treatment of rheumatism because they control the degree of inflammation in the affected joints and it is in the prescribing, changing and altering the dose of these widely differing drugs that the special skill and experience of the Rheumatologist lies.

Aspirin has the unique property of being a useful analgesic drug and when given in larger amounts, ten to twelve 0.3 gm tablets a day in divided doses, has a moderate anti-inflammatory effect, and unless there are any special contra-indications is always the first line of attack. If you take these larger doses you should be warned that dizziness and occasional deafness are not uncommon and the tablets should always be taken with a glass of water, preferably followed by food.

There are many preparations of aspirin some of which have a special coating which diminishes the degree of irritation of the stomach. One preparation which passes through the stomach and which is taken in liquid form and is well tolerated is known as Benoral and Rheumatologists find this is the most acceptable form of aspirin.

During the last few years a whole range of more potent anti-inflammatory drugs has been introduced and among the most effective are Brufen and Indocid. More recently a new anti-inflammatory drug called Feldene has been introduced which it is claimed provides continuous relief of pain and stiffness with a single daily dose. Some people find these drugs give rise to gastric and intestinal upsets and it may be necessary to try several of this group of drugs before finding one to suit a particular individual.

When the joints remain painful and swollen in spite of a thorough trial of these analgesic and anti-inflammatory agents, more powerful drugs are available which have a specific effect on rheumatoid arthritis. These are not suitable for use in cases of osteo-arthritis or spondylitis. They must be taken only under strict supervision, at precise intervals and carefully graduated dosage, and samples of urine tested at frequent intervals. Probably the oldest of these and one which is still used in many hospitals is the injection of gold salts.

Gold

Gold salts were originally used over fifty years ago in the treatment of tuberculosis, and because of the resemblance of T.B. and arthritic joints it was tried in severe cases and found to be effective. It has the disadvantage of having to be injected into muscles and it acts slowly. It is a toxic substance so if you take this drug you must be aware of the danger of adverse reactions, notably skin rashes and a sore mouth. Despite this, if you do not respond to other simpler measures, it may prove to be invaluable. Regular blood and urine tests are necessary while taking gold salts.

Penicillamine

This is a drug related to penicillin which has recently been found to be helpful in the treatment of certain cases of persistent active rheumatoid arthritis which is not responding to the anti-inflammatory drugs. Unlike gold salts it can be taken by mouth but requires careful supervision because of its toxic effects on the blood and kidneys.

Antimalarial drugs

Certain drugs which are useful in the treatment of malaria have been found to have an anti-inflammatory effect in cases of rheumatoid disease but they may cause damage to the retina, and periodic examination of the eye is necessary if the drug is used continuously for many months.

The steroids

We now come to the most powerful and potentially dangerous group of drugs used in the management of cases of rheumatoid arthritis. In order to appreciate their dramatic effect it is necessary to say a few words about hormones.

A hormone is the substance produced by any of the glands of the body which empty directly into the blood stream, e.g. the pancreas produces insulin which controls the level of sugar in the blood, and the thyroid gland produces thyroxin which has a marked effect on the rate of metabolism in the body.

There are two small glands, one lying on the top of each kidney, called the adrenal glands which produce adrenaline – a substance which pours out into the blood stream to assist the body in combating shock.

About fifty years ago research biochemists at the Mayo Clinic isolated several other compounds from the adrenal glands of animals called corticosteroids which they eventually succeeded in making artificially. When sufficient of the drug was available it was given to a man who was crippled with very acute rheumatoid arthritis. Within three days of treatment he was up and about apparently cured. It was soon realised, however, that as soon as the drug was stopped the symptoms reappeared and that it does not cure but only suppresses symptoms. In addition, when used for any length of time unpleasant and often dangerous side-effects appeared.

The skin became thinned and bruised easily, and excessive amounts of fluid were retained in the body with deposits of fat forming particularly around the face and neck causing a round moon-face appearance so that patients taking steroid drugs are easily recognised. Other dangerous complications include softening and collapse of the bones particularly in the weight-bearing areas such as the spine and pelvis, giving rise to spinal deformity and even fractures.

It has also been found that if cortisone is given for long

periods the normal excretion of the adrenal glands gradually diminishes and it takes some time for them to get back to normal. This means that not only will the disease relapse and the arthritic symptoms return but other signs of deficient adrenal excretion will appear, general muscle weakness and a degree of shock. It is particularly important that this should be borne in mind when an operation is contemplated when excess secretion from the adrenal glands is always required. Such patients will require an extra amount of cortisone which is given by injection into the muscles before the anaesthetic is started. This is why steroid cards must be carried by those undergoing this treatment.

Another way of increasing the natural hormones secreted by the adrenal gland is to give an injection of A.C.T.H. The letters stand for adrenal cortex trophic hormone. This is the substance secreted into the blood stream by that remarkable gland situated at the base of the brain known as the pituitary gland and which regulates the activity of all the glands of the body. If A.C.T.H. is injected, the adrenal glands produce more cortisone and the effect is the same as giving cortisone by mouth. It is a useful method of dealing with a sudden aggravation of the disease quickly but for routine use it has the disadvantage of having to be given by injection and is less powerful in its effect than synthetic steroids taken by mouth.

Because steroids are so successful in relieving symptoms in active rheumatoid disease, a great deal of research has been conducted in an effort to find a steroid with potent anti-inflammatory qualities and minimal side-effects. This line of research has not been particularly successful and Prednisolone, one of the oldest preparations and one of the least toxic, is still the steroid of choice.

How are they used?

They should only be used when all other forms of treatment fail to control the disease. They do not replace other forms of treatment but are used as an additional remedy and only in small doses – sufficient to control the symptoms.

The steroids are powerful and dangerous drugs to be taken only under *strict medical supervision* and if you take them you must *always* carry your steroid card with you, giving details of your treatment and the name of the doctor or hospital looking after you, and a supply of tablets.

One of the most effective ways of relieving rheumatic inflammation in joints or neighbouring tendon sheaths is the injection of a local steroid preparation, usually hydro-cortisone, into the painful area. The response is often dramatic, the pain, swelling and inflammation of the joint may settle down in a few hours, enabling graduated exercises and other forms of physical treatment to be started. These injections are given under fully sterile conditions to avoid infection of the joint, and not repeated too frequently as there is some possibility of softening of the underlying bone.

In spite of these rare complications it is a most valuable form of treatment for particular joints which fail to respond to general medical treatment.

It is clear that the whole problem of the treatment of rheumatoid arthritis by drugs is very complicated and has to be carefully adjusted to suit the individual. Pain and swelling of joints may occur in other diseases and a correct diagnosis in the early stage is important before treatment is started. That is why it is so important that medical treatment of rheumatoid arthritis should be supervised throughout by your own doctor and, when necessary, by the specialist in rheumatism at your local hospital. This is not a disease in which self-medication should play any part.

Although you may respond rapidly to treatment in the early stage the disease may flare up from time to time and in some cases permanent damage to various joints occurs. The long continued care of such patients, the necessity to supervise their continued medical treatment and the need to continue research into new forms of treatment has encouraged the development of Arthritic Centres in all the larger hospitals staffed by Rheumatologists.

Research directed to the cause of rheumatoid arthritis is supported and co-ordinated by the Arthritis and Rheumatism Council, a voluntary organisation established to combat the scourge of the rheumatic diseases and which depends on private subscriptions for its funds.

PHYSICAL TREATMENT

So far we have considered the treatment of inflamed rheumatic joints with drugs. What other measures can we use to relieve your pain and swelling? Any inflamed joint will be made worse by exercise, and rest in the acute stage is essential. If several joints are involved, bed rest either at home or if necessary in hospital for two or three weeks is advisable. A warm bed with a comfortable firm mattress and one pillow and analgesic tablets to relieve the pain will result in rapid improvement in your general condition. If you have been having sleepless nights, mild sleeping tablets should be taken for a few nights, but bear in mind the danger of addiction.

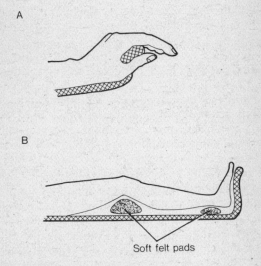

Soft felt pads

Fig. 19.   Some more splints
A   Cock-up splint for wrist.
B   A knee and right angle foot splint.

When resting in bed, care must be taken to avoid deformities of the joints. Your knees must never be kept for long periods in a bent position, and pillows never used to support them. A cradle should be placed at the end of the bed to keep the weight of the bedclothes off painful swollen feet and your head should *not* be pushed forward by using several pillows. When the joints are very swollen light splints may be required to rest the hands, wrists, knees and feet, and these are designed to support the painful joints in the most useful position for use. For example, the fingers are slightly bent, the thumb held in the grasp position and the wrist slightly cocked up. The knees should be straight and the feet supported at a right-angle to the leg. These positions are shown in Fig. 19.

These splints are usually worn for part of the day and often at night during the acute stage of the illness. It is important, however, to learn to contract and relax the muscles which control movement of the joints and with a little practice you can do this at regular intervals without moving the joints at all. This will prevent excessive wasting of the muscles.

Nursing care

When several joints of the upper limb are involved you may feel very helpless and will require help with feeding and special nursing with frequent changes of position if pressure sores are to be avoided. This point is particularly important when you are being treated with cortisone which makes the skin thin, shiny and easily bruised.

Diet

There is no real evidence that special diets have any appreciable effect on rheumatoid disease, except on gout which is a special type of arthritis caused by the formation of excess uric acid in the body because of a faulty metabolism. Patients affected by gout should avoid high protein foods, e.g. "rich meats" like liver, sweetbreads and kidneys.

Otherwise you should have a well-balanced nourishing diet but should avoid eating to excess. With disabled arthritic joints you will probably be able to move around much more easily if you reduce weight.

Alcohol and smoking

Alcohol in moderation is not harmful. The physiological effect of alcohol is to dilate small blood vessels but this may be followed by a secondary contraction, and some rheumatic patients find that it tends to aggravate their pain. Smoking should also be kept to a minimum as nicotine also causes constriction of the small blood vessels. Unfortunately giving up smoking entirely improves the appetite and this may lead to excessive weight. This can affect the heart and certainly makes arthritic joints more troublesome. For some people the best solution is to eat and smoke (for men preferably a pipe) in moderation.

Climate

The effects of climate on rheumatic symptoms have been well studied and two facts emerge The pain and general stiffness is much less in a warm dry climate and is aggravated by exposure to cold damp weather with a falling temperature and barometric pressure. Although the exact reasons are unknown, it is thought to be due to spasm and contraction of the blood vessels which supply the joints and muscles and which occurs in cold weather.

However, a complete change of environment is seldom possible and should certainly not be considered if it involves isolation from friends and relatives with all the possible emotional upset.

Physiotherapy and rehabilitation

Most cases of active rheumatoid arthritis will settle down with adequate rest and possibly splinting of the inflamed joints together with the administration of appropriate drugs. This may take several weeks by which time the muscles may have wasted and the joints stiffened and it is the task of physiotherapists to help you to restore joint mobility and to strengthen the muscles. They will probably have seen you in the acute phase and helped in the application of suitable splints.

As the acute symptoms settle graduated movements and exercises are started. At first the physiotherapist gently puts the joints slowly through a range of movement which can be gradually increased – these are called *passive movements.*

Then you should try to move the joint yourself with some assistance – *assisted active movement.*

Finally you should try to put the joint through a full range of movement, first freely and then against increasing resistance.

ELECTRICAL TREATMENT
Short-wave diathermy

Diathermy is the term used to describe the medical application of high frequency currents. In operating theatres such apparatus is used to coagulate small bleeding vessels.

In the Physiotherapy Department, however, short-wave diathermy is used to apply heat to the deeper tissues of the body by means of an oscillating current of extremely high frequency.

By using insulated pads applied closely to various parts, current flows through the body and the heating effect is produced by the resistance which the deeper structures in the body offer to the current flow.

An insulating pad or a layer of air may be interposed between the electrode and the body surface and this enables a specified region of the body to be heated without undue heating of the skin.

Faradism

Following injury or acutely painful arthritis you sometimes develop a mental inhibition against using the joint at all. The physiotherapist has great difficulty in persuading you to contract the muscles.

In such cases it is often useful to stimulate them by using a faradic current, by means of electrodes applied to skin covering the weakened muscles.

This does *not* mean the mains voltage and is certainly *not* a form of treatment to be used except by a doctor or physiotherapist skilled in its use. The current is produced by using an induction coil and consists of an intermittent alternating current. One electrode covered with a moist cloth is placed in close contact with you and the active electrode, also moistened, is applied to the fleshy part of the muscle and the strength of the current gradually increased. Even in very weak muscles it is possible to produce a strong maintained contracture.

The treatment usually lasts for about fifteen minutes and is continued until you can contract the muscles strongly yourself.

The aim of the physiotherapist is to teach you how, when and how often to practise at home a series of exercises suited to each individual affected joint.

HEAT TREATMENTS

Local heat

Graduated exercises are often more effective if the joints have been warmed up beforehand. Simple measures such as hot towels or hot baths, a gas or electric fire, are often all that is required.

For more regular use radiant heat lamps can be bought for home use at a chemist's. They give out infra-red heat rays. The instructions for use will accompany the lamp – but in general they are usually directed at the painful area, about three feet away, and applied for ten to fifteen minutes.

Hot packs

Since time immemorial various heated solids have been applied to painful regions of the body. Hot salt or sand bags, hot irons and bricks have been used, but have largely been supplanted by other forms of heat, more easily applied and controlled.

Hot mud packs, however, are still used, particularly in continental spas, and claims are made that they have special curative properties. There is no convincing evidence that they contain any radio-active or other specific remedy and it would seem that there are no particular advantages over simpler and cleaner methods of local application of heat.

Hot paraffin wax packs

Hot paraffin wax is a clean and effective agent for raising the temperature of a localised region of the body and is particularly useful for the painful stiff hand and fingers. Ordinary paraffin wax like that used to seal preserving jars is melted in a double boiler to approx. 75°C, which is the low melting point of paraffin. It is allowed to cool a little, and the temperature tested before the wax is painted on in successive layers over the painful area. A hand or foot can be dipped in the paraffin about six times and the heavy covering of paraffin will retain its own heat for a long time and it can then be easily peeled off and reheated and used many times again.

Contrast bathing is also helpful before practising exercises. Hot and cold showers or soaking the part to be exercised for two minutes alternately in hot and cold water will help to stimulate the circulation and should be continued for about ten minutes. In the early stages when your joint is swollen and painful, simple muscle contractions should be practised with little or no movement of the joint. This is particularly important in the knee joint where the muscles in front of the thigh tend to waste rapidly. This particular exercise is known as quadriceps drill and you should practise it for five minutes every hour of the day. The muscle is tightened and kept tight for about thirty seconds and then allowed to relax.

EXERCISES

As the swelling settles down, start active exercises, first with the aid of gravity, then with a sling and finally against gravity and resistance.

The purpose of these exercises is to regain as much movement as possible in the arthritic joint without causing it to flare up. If you are too energetic at the start, the joint may become more painful, tender and swollen. So the movement should be performed slowly and deliberately, trying to coax it a little further each time. Pain and stiffness after exercises means that they have been too strenuous or continued for too long. Some discomfort in the later stages of treatment is inevitable and must be accepted when trying to restore full function to the joint. You will quickly learn how much the joint will stand without too much reaction.

EXERCISES IN GENERAL
Foot and ankle:
Circular movements of the feet clockwise and anti-clockwise (Fig. 20 A). Splay the toes and curl them over a rail. Bend the feet up and down (Fig. 20 B).

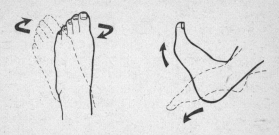

Fig. 20. Foot and ankle exercises
    A Circular movement of the foot clockwise and anti-clockwise.
    B Bending the foot up and down.

The knee:

Tighten the thigh muscles by straightening the knee from a relaxed position (Fig. 21 A). Lift the straight leg from the horizontal. Bicycling exercises when lying on the back (Fig. 21 B).

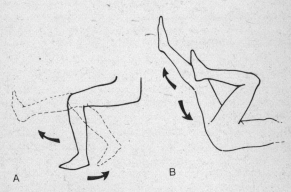

Fig. 21. Knee exercises
    A Tightening the thigh muscles by straightening and bending the knee from a relaxed position.
    B Bicycling exercises when lying on the back.

The hip:

Full rotation movements when lying on back. Circular movements with knee bent on the chest (Fig. 22A). Raise the leg up, out and across, and backward when lying on side (Fig. 22 B).

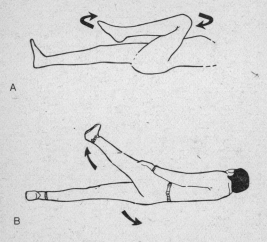

Fig. 22.   Hip exercises
   A   Circular movement with knee bent on to chest.
   B   Raising the leg up, out and across, and backwards when lying on side.

The shoulder:

Start with pendulum exercises practised while leaning forward and tilting towards the affected side (Fig. 23 A). Then practise lifting the arm from the side to the horizontal position and across the opposite shoulder (fig. 23 B), then behind the neck (Fig. 23 C) and finally behind the back trying to reach as high as possible (Fig. 23 D).

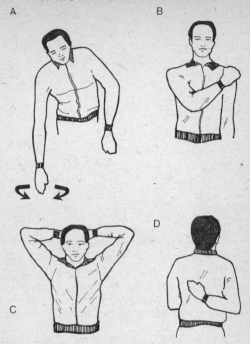

Fig. 23.   Shoulder exercises
  A   Pendulum exercises.
  B   Lifting an arm to horizontal and across to opposite shoulder.
  C   Arms behind the neck.
  D   Reaching up as high as possible behind the back.

Elbow and wrist:

Bend and straighten both joints and particularly stress rotation movements of the forearm bones.

Fingers:

The fingers should be exercised continuously by carrying round a hard sponge rubber ball and gripping it firmly and frequently.

5

RHEUMATISM IN CHILDREN

Children often complain of aches which come and go, particularly in their legs. Sometimes these are related to exercise – a strenuous game of football or training for competitive running and are probably due to minor strains of muscles and tendons which clear up with a period of rest from vigorous games.

Others appear to have no obvious cause and we often call them "growing pains" for lack of any real explanation. Sometimes the child is merely seeking attention – like "the glass of water" at night - and it is very common for young children to mimic their parents' complaints and limps. Most children grow out of this stage but if the complaints persist you should not dismiss them completely without some investigation and particularly if the affected joint appears swollen or the painful area is tender. In such cases a visit to your doctor is advisable who will if necessary arrange for X-rays and a blood test to exclude a bone injury or some infection.

Sometimes an intermittent limp with pain in the knee may indicate mild inflammation of the hip, the so-called transient synovitis of the hip or a disturbance of the normal growth of the upper end of the femur which we call Perthe's disease.

Small children frequently fall over when playing unobserved and may sustain slight crack fractures of the bones of the leg which do not prevent them from walking but cause pain and a limp. Occasionally pains in the limbs have a psychological explanation – a manifestation of some unhappiness or sense of insecurity or fear of bullying at school.

These are some of the minor causes of pain in the limbs in

children and if an organic cause has been excluded they will settle down with reassurance and occasional periods of rest. It is important that the symptoms should not be over-emphasised and that an over-protective attitude is avoided. Occasionally, however, children do suffer from more serious forms of arthritis.

RHEUMATIC FEVER

Fifty years ago rheumatic fever was one of the commonest and most serious diseases of childhood. Nowadays in Britain and the Western World it is rare and when it occurs is a comparatively mild disease, although it is still frequently seen in poorer countries, with problems of overcrowding and malnutrition.

This is a particular type of acute rheumatism which affects mainly children between the age of five to fifteen years. It starts with a severe sore throat and a throat swab shows that the infecting germ is a type known as a streptococcus. As this particular germ is readily sensitive to a range of antibiotics the throat infection can be quickly cured and rheumatic fever is nowadays a rare condition.

It is diagnosed during the course of an acute throat infection by the sudden onset of a persistently high temperature and pain and swelling of one or more joints. Several joints may be involved and the pain flits from one joint to another. No permanent damage to the joint occurs but a small proportion of children will develop heart disease due to a rheumatic inflammation of the heart muscles and the formation of nodules on the heart valves.

Other signs of the disease are skin rashes, painless nodules under the skin, and some children develop a nervous muscle twitching known as chorea or St. Vitus' dance. Rheumatic fever is a serious condition but it responds very well to treatment with penicillin. Because the attacks are likely to recur with each new throat infection these must be treated promptly with penicillin and it may be necessary to continue with antibiotics for several years. When teeth are extracted bacteria may gain entrance to the blood stream and penicillin must be given before dental treatment is started.

During the acute stage of the illness the joint symptoms settle down well when treated with large doses of aspirin, and if the heart is damaged treatment with special drugs for the heart, e.g. digoxin, may be required later. Narrowing of the heart valves is a possible complication of rheumatic fever and nowadays this can be treated by heart surgery if it is serious.

JUVENILE ARTHRITIS (STILL'S DISEASE)

Dr. Still, a physician at Great Ormond Street Hospital, London, was the first doctor to describe a more chronic form of arthritis in children which in many respects resembles rheumatoid arthritis in adults.

It is a rare and in most cases a mild disease, which usually clears up completely, but very occasionally continues into adult life with crippling deformities.

The first sign of the disease is usually some swelling of the knees or wrists which may take a long time to settle down and may recur from time to time. There is very little pain and usually little evidence of inflammation of the joints, but occasionally the child may be feverish, generally out of sorts, with swollen glands, inflamed eyes and a rash.

In children the growing end of a long bone forms part of the joint which is inflamed in rheumatism. The effect of this inflammation is first of all to stimulate the growth of bones but later in the disease the bones may fail to grow and shortening or deformities such as knock-knee may result.

TREATMENT

Treatment is very similar to the treatment of rheumatoid arthritis in adults. In the acute stage the child may need adequate rest but need not be confined to bed entirely. The inflamed joints may require supporting with light splints which can be easily removed for passive movements and gentle exercises in warm water or, if available, a pool. The type of drugs used will vary according to the severity of the disease. In mild cases aspirin will suffice but more severe cases may require gold injections or cortisone. More severe cases will require to be in hospital for special schooling and more intensive physiotherapy but these periods should be kept to a minimum provided the home conditions are satisfactory. A disabled child does need considerable attention and this may not be possible if there are several children to be looked after.

Very rarely some form of surgery may be required to correct deformities or to replace a badly damaged joint with an artificial one. In time the active disease settles down and modern orthopaedic treatment will enable even the very crippled child to lead a reasonably active life. There is no evidence that this disease is hereditary and there need be no anxiety about their passing the disease on to their children.

6

OSTEO-ARTHRITIS

This is the commonest form of arthritis. The characteristic feature is the formation of bony spurs or bumps around the margin of a joint - hence the prefix osteo - which means bone. Because it is an ageing or wear-and-tear process of a joint and not an inflammation, the suffix "itis" is not really applicable and medical purists tend to call it osteo-arthrosis.

The changes which occur in the joint are first seen in the cartilage covering the bone-ends. The cartilage cells become swollen and begin to degenerate and cracks appear in the smooth cartilage surface, which gradually wears away with continued use. Over a period of years loss of the normal smooth gliding surface gives rise to instability of the joint and nature's defence is to lay down new calcified bone around the edges of the joint – a hard bony rim which can often be seen and felt in joints in old people – particularly the finger joints.

Loss of the smooth articular cartilage gives rise to stiffness of the joint and occasionally bits of bone or cartilage break away and lie loose in the joint causing sudden pain and a locking sensation. To some extent this is a natural ageing process which in varying degrees affects all tissues of the body. Some people age more quickly than others; the weight-bearing joints may tend to wear at a younger age and this tendency may be hereditary.

Professional sportsmen, such as footballers and long distance runners, put excessive stress on the hips, knees and ankles over many years and are more liable to develop osteo-arthritis of these joints in middle age.

Other factors play their part. A single severe injury to a joint, repeated minor strains or abnormal positions maintained for long periods, e.g. the fully squatting position in a miner working on a low seam, are all factors which may result in progressive osteo-arthritis.

Osteo-arthritis is a slow insidious disorder usually starting in late middle age. The arthritic changes in the joint as seen on an X-ray are often severe before the joint becomes painful because neither the new bone formed nor the worn cartilage have many pain sensitive nerve endings. The earliest symptom is stiffness of the joint, particularly in the morning after lying in bed, or sitting for long periods in a car or theatre. When the bony spurs begin to press on sensitive tissues such as the synovial membrane, or joint capsule, or the ligaments, and muscles are strained, the joint becomes painful. This is worse in cold damp weather because the small blood vessels which supply these structures become constricted.

The joints which bear the weight of the body, the hips, knees and the spine are more commonly affected, particularly if used to excess or they have to carry too much weight and a common story is that people approaching middle age, who put on weight, find they are unable to walk as fast or as far as they could and have increasing difficulty in keeping up their sporting activities.

Osteo-arthritis may come on at a younger age in joints which have never been quite normal, and children suffering from congenital dislocation of the hip may be left with a joint in which the upper end of the femur and the socket do not fit properly and the cartilage wears out more rapidly.

Perthe's disease of the hip in children is a condition in which there is some interference with the normal growth of the head of the femur and this again may result in an incongruous joint with pain and stiffness in later years. However, if both these conditions are discovered and treated at an early stage the hip joint will grow normally and trouble in later life can be avoided.

TREATMENT OF OSTEO-ARTHRITIS

The bones and articular cartilages are the tissues primarily involved in osteo-arthritis but it is the associated inflammation in the synovial membrane and capsule of the joints which cause pain. Excessive use of the joint, increased weight and exposure to cold and wet conditions aggravate the pain. Avoiding strenuous activities, and particularly dieting are important factors in easing symptoms. In addition, measures to improve the circulation of the joint, e.g. various forms of heat and graduated exercise, are helpful.

Diet

There is no particular diet which will cure arthritis, but some people do find that they are allergic to certain foods, e.g. citrus fruits may make their symptoms worse and they should be avoided.

Osteo-arthritis usually affects older people and when the weight-bearing joints are involved, e.g. the hip, knee or ankle, they have to lead a more sedentary life and will inevitably put on weight. Thus a vicious circle is set up as the excess weight makes these joints more painful.

Keeping weight down is probably the most important factor in relieving the chronic ache of an osteo-arthritic joint. Everyone can reduce weight by sticking to a reasonable diet but some people put on weight more easily than others.

On a well-balanced diet of 1,400 calories most people should be able to lose 8 lbs to 10 lbs a month and all arthritic centres attached to hospitals work closely with dieticians who will advise on a variety of suitable diets which can be both tasty and interesting. Self-discipline is the clue to successful dieting. Never over-eat and avoid sugar, cut down carbohydrates and pastries and eat plenty of protein, e.g. fish.

Physiotherapy

Hospital Physiotherapy Departments are usually hard pressed and it is important that their limited resources are used to the best advantage. A programme of treatment is planned and emphasis is placed on teaching you to help yourself by performing carefully graduated exercises at home. Local heat to the joint by means of an infra-red lamp or short-wave diathermy followed by a course of exercises, assisted at first but later progressing to exercises against resistance, are followed by more strenuous physical exercises in a group.

The other important function of the physiotherapist is to keep up your morale. You must clearly understand that osteo-arthritis is not a generalised disease like rheumatoid arthritis and on the whole has a much better outlook. Although pain and stiffness of the hip and knee can cause considerable disability, the symptoms will improve with treatment and many cases may be permanently relieved.

Sometimes, however, the joints gradually become more painful and the disability slowly increases with progressive stiffness and lameness. Nevertheless the recent developments in the surgical treatment of painful arthritic joints may provide dramatic improvement in activity.

Home treatment

Much of the treatment that is carried out in an expensive spa or hospital Physiotherapy Department can be done at home with simple measures. The easiest way to apply heat to arthritic joints is to soak in a hot bath or apply moist heat by means of a towel rung out in hot water. These compresses should be applied for fifteen minutes two or three times a day just above body temperature.

Other forms of heat which are readily available at home are the electric radiator or electric pad or blanket, and a deeper form of heat can be provided by using infra-red lamps which are readily available at the chemist and can be plugged into an ordinary electric socket.

Another useful method of applying heat, particularly to the hands, is to soak in warm paraffin wax when the heat is retained for some time. After the joint has been thoroughly heated, massage the painful area away from the dependent part of the limb with powder or cream and begin graduated exercises. These should be started in a hot bath when the buoyancy of the water will assist movements. They should be performed slowly, aiming to put the stiffened joint through as full a range of movement as possible, and then trying to coax it a little further. In addition to attempting to increase movement the exercises are also aimed at strengthening the muscles. These should be carried out regularly, morning and evening, and at intervals three or four times during the day, at first with the assistance of gravity, then against gravity, and later against strong resistance. More vigorous weight-bearing exercises are used when the condition is improving.

Some temporary reaction in the way of increased swelling and stiffness after exercise often occurs. If it persists the treatment has probably been too strenuous and the time spent on exercise should be reduced.

Contrast bathing

This is particularly applicable to arthritic changes in the foot or ankle and helps to stimulate the circulation before mobilising exercises. Using either a shower or bowls of water, the affected joints are soaked alternately in hot and cold water for two minutes at a time for a period of about ten minutes.

Other preventive measures

The chronic aches and pains associated with increasing age and early degenerative joint changes are often aggravated by working in an uncomfortable position for long periods, sleeping in a slumped position on a soft mattress, driving a car for long periods with an ill-adjusted seat or steering wheel or a stiff clutch pedal. A firm mattress and using only one pillow, adjusting the height of an office desk or chair, and a support to the back when driving are all examples of simple measures which may well help an aching back or neck. The author can vouch for the fact that driving a car with automatic gears is a great help when suffering from trouble with the left hip or knee.

Body posture

As one gets older it becomes increasingly important to control consciously the natural tendency of the body to "slump". This is a position adopted when we are tired when we rely on the inactive ligaments to support the body and this puts an undue strain on the joints so that we gradually acquire a permanent round back, sagging belly and walk with a shuffling gait with feet turned out.

Mr. W. E. Tucker has for some years stressed the importance of acquiring what he describes as an active alerted posture. This is achieved by gripping the floor with the toes and turning the feet inwards a little with the knees slightly bent. Tighten the muscles of the stomach wall and the buttocks, raise the shoulders slightly and tuck the chin in. He describes it vividly as preparation for action.[1]

"(1) Stand like a successful bow-legged jockey not like a knock-kneed flat-footed tramp.

(2) Stand with a rock bottom and pinch proof posterior instead of a sagging back with a prominent belly.

(3) Stand as if the top of your head were linked to a star, instead of with the rounded sloping shoulders of a beggar."

Drugs

Simple analgesic or pain-relieving drugs are often all that are required in osteo-arthritis, and the most useful is aspirin which has in addition an anti-inflammatory action. Because it has an irritant effect on the stomach, aspirin, or to give it its chemical name acetyl salicylic acid, may be combined with other drugs, e.g. bufferin, to neutralise the stomach acid, or tablets may be coated to prevent their being dissolved in the stomach and pass on to be digested in the intestines. The drug Benoral is probably the least irritant form of aspirin. Because there is always a degree of local joint inflammation in osteo-arthritis some of the anti-inflammatory drugs more commonly used in rheumatoid arthritis may be effective. Among the most useful are Indocid, Brufen and Feldene, and any of these drugs may be prescribed with the usual precaution that unusual side-effects such as dizziness, nausea or headache must be reported immediately.

Steroid drugs

The steroid drugs should never be given by mouth in osteo-arthritis but they are often helpful when injected locally into the joint or the ligaments or capsule. 5 cc of hydrocortisone injected into a swollen painful joint will often result in dramatic improvement and may be repeated at intervals of a

[1] From "Home Treatment and Posture", by W. E. Tucker, published by Churchill Livingstone, Edinburgh.

month. They should not be used on more than three or four occasions because of the danger of causing further degeneration to the articular cartilage.

Manipulation and local anaesthesia

In the early stages of arthritis stiffness and pain on certain movements localised to a particular spot may be the main symptoms. In such cases relief is obtained by an injection of a local anaesthetic into the painful area followed by manipulations of the joint to increase the range of movement. These are the sort of cases which are often improved or "cured" by the bone-setter or osteopath. This form of treatment is, however, readily available at all major arthritic centres after full medical and X-ray investigations have been carried out.

7

SURGICAL TREATMENT OF OSTEO-ARTHRITIS

Probably the biggest advances in the treatment of arthritic conditions in recent years have resulted from the surgical treatment of very disorganised joints and this applies particularly to the painful osteo-arthritic hip.

MINOR OPERATIONS

Neuritis

The thickening of ligaments and capsule around an arthritic joint may cause pressure on nerves lying close to the joint and cause tingling and numbness. This occurs occasionally around the elbow joint but more commonly the wrist, and a small operation to free the nerve usually clears up the symptoms.

Cysts

Soft swellings may develop around affected joints due to leaking of excess synovial fluid escaping into the surrounding tissues and forming cysts. These may enlarge and become painful and if necessary can be removed.

TRIGGER FINGERS

The tendons which move across an arthritic joint may become trapped and fail to glide smoothly. This occurs more frequently around the wrist and fingers and results in limitation of movement or a painful snapping sensation when using the fingers. This can be relieved quite easily by opening up the constricted tendon sheath.

SYNOVECTOMY

When an arthritic joint becomes chronically swollen and has not responded to drugs and physical treatment, including aspirations and injections of hydrocortisone, the inflamed synovial membrane slowly destroys the articular cartilage. The surgeon may advise an operation to remove as much of the joint lining as possible. This diminishes the secretion of excess fluid and a more normal joint lining re-forms. This operation is more commonly performed for intractable arthritis of the knee joint and is known as a synovectomy.

OSTEOTOMY

Many cases of osteo-arthritis of the hip and knee are associated with some deformity of the leg - a flexion deformity

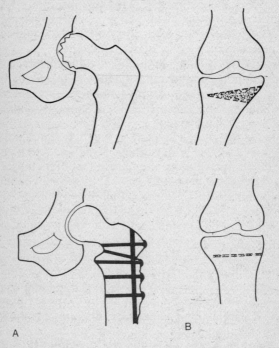

A

B

Fig. 24. Osteotomy
A   Osteotomy to correct flexion deformities of the hip by straightening the bone, and
B   To correct bowing or knock-knee deformities of the knee.

of the hip joint, or bowing or knock-knee deformity at the knee joint, and the operation to correct these deformities is known as an osteotomy. The bone or bones adjacent to the joints are divided and fixed in correct alignment by a metal plate, as shown in Fig. 24. When the bone is soundly healed the joint will function more normally and a good deal of the pain will be relieved.

ARTHROPLASTY

This is an operation to form a new joint. When the joint is completely destroyed by the arthritic process, removal of the bone ends and the worn-out cartilage covering is followed by the growth of fibrous tissue between the cut surfaces and a degree of painless movement, although with some instability, may be achieved.

The operation is sometimes used to restore movement to stiff painful toe joints, the elbow joint and, occasionally when all else fails, the hip joint. It is known as an excision arthroplasty.

TOTAL ARTHROPLASTY OR TOTAL JOINT REPLACEMENT

This is the operation which has been developed so successfully during recent years in the case of the hip joint and more recently the knee.

There are many modifications of this procedure. Basically they consist of removing the articulating bone ends and adjacent cartilage. In the case of the hip, the socket in the pelvis and the upper end or head of the femur are removed and replaced by a plastic cup made of high density polyethylene, and a stainless steel component for the upper end of the femur (Fig. 25 A). These are firmly fixed in position by bone cement.

The results of this operation are in the majority of cases excellent with a very good chance of walking painlessly for many years.

Replacement arthroplasty of the knee joint (Fig. 25 B) is technically more difficult and there is less chance of achieving a painless stable joint.

The technical difficulties of replacing painful arthritic shoulder and elbow joints are gradually being overcome, and

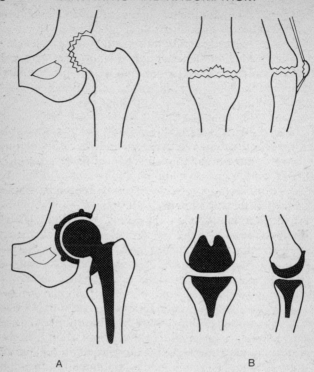

Fig. 25. **Arthroplasty**
  A Total replacement of the hip when the joint cartilage is very worn and irregular.
  B Total replacement of the knee joint in similar circumstances.

finger and toe joints have been replaced with varying degrees of success. Severely painful and deformed joints can be successfully treated by replacing them with malleable plastic joints correcting the deformity at the same time.

ARTHRODESIS

Before the introduction of replacement arthroplasties patients with a completely disorganised painful joint were often better off if the joint was made stiff and the operation to fix joints is known as an arthrodesis.

Although some disability was inevitable pain was relieved completely and provided the neighbouring joints were mobile the patients often walked surprisingly well in spite of a stiff hip or knee.

INDICATIONS FOR SURGERY

The decision as to whether an operation is advisable in treating arthritic joints is never easy and it is essential for you to be fully informed about the chances of success and the possible risks of any procedure.

You, in turn, must carefully assess the degree of pain and disability from which you are suffering.

An intermittent ache and the necessity to use a stick when walking any distance are not disabilities requiring surgery and operations are only considered when suffering intractable pain unrelieved by analgesics and physical treatment, particularly if sleep is constantly interrupted. Replacement arthroplasty of the hip is particularly successful in restoring almost normal function to a stiff deformed joint but it is a major operation with a small but significant rate of complications. You should bear this possibility, however remote, in mind. Clotting of the big veins of the leg, infection of the wound and loosening of the components of the joint all occur in a small percentage of cases but if the alternative is a life of serious invalidism these are risks worth taking.

The sensible plan is to discuss the matter with relatives and the family doctor and then consult a surgeon familiar with these operations, but the ultimate decision rests with you. Never be too influenced by other people who have had replacement operations because no two cases are identical and some joints are more difficult to restore than others.

8

GOUT

This disease is a form of arthritis characterised by sudden attacks of acute pain, swelling and inflammation of various joints - one of the commonest to be involved is the big toe joint. It was the first arthritic condition to be described centuries ago, and traditionally affected the wealthier sections of the community, who tended to lead sedentary lives and eat food rich in proteins. Among its famous victims were Harvey, the discoverer of the circulation of the blood, George IV and William Pitt.

Metabolism is the process by which the body changes the food we eat and the oxygen we breathe into proteins, carbohydrates and fat. These are used to build up new tissues and eliminate waste products. Gout is a metabolic disease in which something has gone wrong with this mechanism.

Among the waste products which are formed in the body are substances called purines and when these are broken down they form uric acid. This circulates in the blood and is partly excreted in the kidneys to form one of the acid components of the urine.

If you have gout, uric acid is formed in greater quantities, resulting in an excessive amount circulating in the blood, and in an attempt to get rid of this excess it is deposited in crystal form in various joints, in cartilages and other organs.

We do not know why some people have this inborn error of metabolism but the disease is hereditary and is commoner in men over forty.

Over-eating is not the cause of gout. However, indulging particularly in rich meats such as liver, brain or sweetbreads which contain an excess of purines, or too much alcohol, notably heavy wines or port, will often bring on an attack. Cold and damp weather and emotional stress are other factors which may play a part in the onset. Sufferers from gout are prone to attacks after an operation and should always inform the surgeon of this beforehand. A minor injury to a joint may also bring on an attack or be responsible for the pain persisting.

In a typical attack the affected joints swell rapidly, become warm and red and very tender so that even the pressure of bedclothes cannot be tolerated. These attacks may last for a week or two and are often accompanied by some fever and may recur for long intervals, often months or years. Occasionally they are more frequent when the joints become permanently enlarged and deformed.

The crystals may collect in tissues other than joints - common sites are the edges of the ears and behind the elbow where they form firm chalky swellings called "tophi", or the kidneys, giving rise to kidney stones.

When gout is suspected a simple blood test to measure the amount of uric acid in the blood will establish the diagnosis and is also useful in estimating the effect of treatment.

TREATMENT

In contrast to rheumatoid arthritis the modern treatment of gout is reliable and quickly effective and permanent damage to joints which was a common feature of the disease in the past can now be avoided.

Diet

Food rich in purines, e.g. liver, kidney, sweetbreads, etc., must be avoided completely and meat also eaten in moderation. Alcohol particularly may precipitate an attack – heavy red wines and beer are better avoided. Dilute whisky and gin are less harmful.

The acute attack

It is important to commence treatment as soon as the attack starts so if you are a chronic sufferer you should have the appropriate tablets available immediately. The most effective drug is a very old remedy called colchicine. Two tablets should be taken at the start of the attack and an additional tablet every hour throughout the day until the pain is relieved up to a total of six to eight tablets a day. Occasionally this drug causes nausea and diarrhoea and some doctors may prefer to prescribe Butazolidin or Indocid, the drugs which are frequently used in the treatment of rheumatoid arthritis.

Preventive treatment

If the attacks become frequent it may prove necessary to take drugs during the interval between attacks to get rid of excess uric acid in the system. Some of these drugs help to flush out uric acid through the kidneys while others, e.g. Allopurinol, reduce the amount of uric acid the body makes.

General measures

During the acute attack you should rest and cold moist compresses or ice packs applied to the inflamed joint may help to diminish the swelling and ease the pain. Gout is one arthritic disorder which responds quickly to treatment. Medical advice should be obtained early in the disease and carefully followed. With strict attention to diet you should be able to lead a normal vigorous life.

9

THE PAINFUL NECK

Pain in the neck is one of the commonest and most troublesome symptoms affecting people in middle age. Although often no more than a mild inconvenience, it *may* be severe and incapacitating.

Anatomy

The seven bones of the neck resemble those of the rest of the spine but their shape is adapted to provide support to the skull, and movement, enabling you to turn your head round freely in all directions.

As in the lumbar region these cervical vertebrae are separated by pads of cartilage or discs. Between the vertebrae, in close contact with the discs, are two holes through which the spinal nerves pass from the spinal cord down to the arms. the vertebrae are held together by strong ligaments and movement is controlled by a number of powerful muscles.

CAUSES OF NECK PAIN

Fibrositis

As in other parts of the spine pain and stiffness may be caused by a mild inflammation of the muscles or ligaments which we call fibrositis – the result of minor strains of the neck and aggravated by sudden changes in temperature from sitting in a cold damp draught. These symptoms usually settle down in a few days. Prolonged poor posture, as when sitting at a low desk or sleeping heavily with too many pillows, may also give rise to pain and stiffness of the neck.

Injury

One of the commonest causes of intractable pain in the neck

results from damage to the disc and ligaments in a car collision. The body of the driver or passenger is held back by a seat belt or sudden bracing against the dashboard while the head is thown rapidly forward and then jerked back. This is known as a *whip-lash injury* and may cause prolonged pain and stiffness in the neck, the pain often radiating down the arms. This type of injury can be avoided or at least minimised by the use of head rests in cars.

More severe injuries to the head and neck may result in damage to the cartilage discs which become flattened and broader giving rise to pressure on one of the spinal nerves. This causes pain not only on neck movement but also pain radiating down into the shoulder and arm, and in very severe injuries the damaged disc may cause pressure on the spinal cord with varying degrees of paralysis.

Wear and tear

Over the years the small joints of the neck and the discs slowly degenerate. They become narrowed with thickened bony margins called osteophytes which limit neck movements causing stiffness and pressure on the spinal nerves. This condition is called *cervical spondylosis* and is present in most people after the age of forty and may be responsible for repeated attacks of pain and stiffness in the neck.

Arthritis of the cervical spine

Rheumatoid arthritis may involve every joint of the body and the small joints of the neck are commonly involved. Neck movements become progressively limited and the nerve roots may be pressed on by damage to the vertebrae or stretched when the softened ligaments allow the bones of the neck to become displaced. Either way pain radiates from the neck down the arm and movement of the head and neck aggravates the pain.

Similarly osteo-arthritis may involve the joints of the neck in older people resulting in stiffness and pain on movement. This is particularly severe in ankylosing spondylitis (see page 37). This condition starts with aching and stiffness of the lower part of the back and spreads to involve the throracic spine and finally the neck. In severe cases it may produce almost complete rigidity of the head and neck and the head may become fixed with the neck in a bent position so that the victim of this rare but sometimes serious disease may look permanently downwards at his feet.

THE SYMPTOMS

"Creaking"

The neck is very near the inner ear and you may hear creaks and clicks on moving your neck. This is caused by thickened ligaments or roughened bones moving on each other and is more severe in arthritis of the neck.

Neck ache

In addition to pain on movement, a dull ache may result from muscular effort to support and hold your head still. The pain is often felt in the back of the head or may radiate over your shoulders and down your arms and may be accompanied by tingling in your fingers. These symptoms are often troublesome at night and are made worse by sleeping with the head in an abnormal position – the result of using too many pillows and sleeping on a soft mattress.

TREATMENT

Home Treatment

Many stiff painful necks will settle down with local heat from a hot water bottle or radiator, together with gentle massage to your neck and shoulder muscles, and simple pain-relieving tablets such as aspirin or distalgesics. If these attacks recur frequently you should consult your doctor who will arrange for X-rays to be taken to exclude any signs of arthritis of the cervical spine.

Collars

Supporting the neck in some sort of collar will often relieve a persistent ache in your neck or pain radiating to your shoulders. Collars can be made at home from a folded newspaper or a thick layer of felt wrapped in a scarf and covered with a stocking. This will provide warmth and support to your head and restrict neck movement.

For intractable pain associated with severe arthritis or disease or injury to the bones of the neck, more rigid types of collar made of new materials (which can be moulded when heated) are available from hospital appliance makers.

Traction, manipulation and exercises

Some cases of neck pain prove very intractable but may respond to traction and skilled manipulation. This form of treatment should only be used after the condition has been fully investigated and the neck X-rayed and then only by doctors, physiotherapists or osteopaths who have been fully trained and are experienced in this technique. The traction is applied by firmly grasping your head and pulling slowly and steadily stretching your neck. When your neck muscles are relaxed your head is gently manipulated in various directions to free any adhesions which may have formed around the joints or to correct minor displacements.

Vigorous sudden movements must be avoided as they may cause damage to your spinal cord.

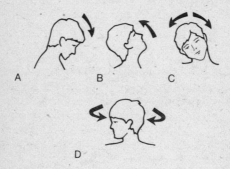

Fig. 26.   Neck exercises
    A   Flexion.
    B   Extension.
    C   Tilting.
    D   Rotation.

A more gradual method of applying traction is by means of a harness applied to your head and another to your trunk. Slow distraction (pulling apart) of the neck can then be produced mechanically and this may free the nerves from pressure. Once the pain has been relieved exercises will help to get rid of stiffness and strengthen your neck muscles. Fig. 26 shows different ways of putting the joints of the neck through as full a range of movement as possible.

10

THE PAINFUL FOOT

There are a large number of joints in your foot, any one of which may be affected by arthritis – either rheumatoid arthritis or the wear and tear of osteo-arthritis. These small joints carry a great deal of weight for long periods and the ligaments which join them together are under constant strain.

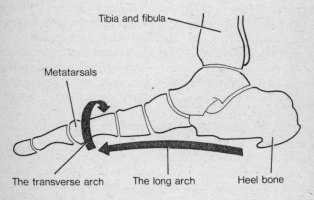

Fig. 27.   The foot
Illustrating the arches.

The arches of the foot

There are two arches to your foot. One runs the length of your foot from your heel to the base of your toes and a smaller, lower transverse arch supports the metatarsal heads. These arches are maintained by muscles and ligaments and provide a springy cushion which absorbs the sudden pressure on the sole of your foot when walking, running or jumping. The heights of these arches vary considerably from one person to another. Some people have a very low arch and others a high arch but it is not the height of the arch which is important. It is whether your feet are supple and bones move easily one on the other.

The nutrition of the foot

The feet are like the hands – sensitive structures – and when injured or the site of arthritis can be very painful. They are also at the end of the path of circulation of the blood and when this fails, as it often does in old people, the feet are often the first to suffer. Poor circulation of the feet gives rise to a severe burning pain and the skin easily becomes ulcerated, particularly in sufferers from diabetes.

These symptoms of pain, numbness and ulceration of the feet or toes are often thought to be due to arthritis. While some arthritic changes may well be present in the joints of your toes and feet it is important to find out whether the circulation is impaired and particularly whether diabetes is present.

This is why it is so important when such symptoms develop to consult your doctor who can decide by a simple examination of the circulation and urine test whether these disorders are present and can start appropriate treatment.

DEFORMITIES OF THE FOOT AND TOES

Shoes and socks

Ill-fitting shoes and tight socks worn for long periods during the period of rapid growth, five to 14 years, are the commonest cause of painful deformities of the feet and toes in later life.

The problem is worse with girls because they do not wear their shoes out as quickly as boys and thus tend to wear them longer, and fashion dictates that their shoes should be narrow fitting, the toes pointed and the heels abnormally high. The effect is to crowd the toes by pushing the forepart of the foot into the narrow pointed part of the shoe.

Worn for limited periods these cause little harm but if worn more or less continuously the toes become squashed together and in their late 'teens girls may develop the following deformities:

1.   *A bunion* – here the big toe deviates outwards and a bony bump develops on the inner side of the big toe joint which is painful and may become inflamed.

2.   *A rigid big toe joint*. Continued pressure on the end of the big toes gradually wears out the cartilage covering the bones of the big toe joint which become stiff and painful on walking.

3.   *A hammer toe*. This deformity usually affects the second toe. Because they are unable to lie flat when the shoe is too tight, the toes tend to buckle at the joints between the first and second bones of the toes, resulting in a fixed bony deformity of the toe which is constantly pressed on and irritated by the pressure of the shoe. The first joint of the toe is bent up and the top of the joint is pressed into the toe-cap producing a painful pressure sore. When both the joints of the toes are bent and the toes curled down we describe the deformity as claw toes. This can be a particularly troublesome deformity causing pain over the top of toes and the transverse arch of the foot is pushed down resulting in a painful callosity under the forefoot.

THE FEET IN RHEUMATOID ARTHRITIS

Pain in the feet is sometimes the first symptom of rheumatoid arthritis. The metatarsal phalangeal joints, the joints between the fore part of your foot and your toes, become swollen and tender, the ligaments slacken and the arches drop and the forefoot spreads. Your toes develop hammer toe deformities and your big toe is pushed outwards and a bunion develops which may ulcerate and become inflamed.

It is important before toe deformities are treated to make sure there is no evidence of active disease. This can be done by X-ray examination which will show the characteristic eroded areas in your bones near the joints and a blood test which will demonstrate whether the disease is active and you require treatment for rheumatoid arthritis. It is no use embarking on surgical treatment for deformities if the disease is in a very active phase.

TREATMENT OF DEFORMITIES OF THE FOOT AND TOES

Deformity alone is seldom an indication for surgical

treatment. If your feet and toes are completely mobile they are seldom painful.

Most of the discomfort is due to a rigid deformity with pressure of the shoe on protuberant bones.

In older people with very deformed feet and particularly in the presence of arthritis of the joints, specially adapted shoes are essential and may be all that is required. They must be light and roomy with soft uppers and fitting the contour of the foot, and the soles must be reasonably pliable. A sponge rubber insole covered with soft leather may be required to support the long arch of your foot and relieve the forefoot of undue pressure. These shoes have to be specially made and are expensive but in the U.K. can be obtained under the National Health Service at reduced cost.

Surgical treatment

In younger people without any active disease the painful protruding bones can successfully be removed and the toes straightened by a variety of operations. However, if you embark on any foot or toe operations you should appreciate that they are not minor procedures from which recovery can be expected in a week or two.

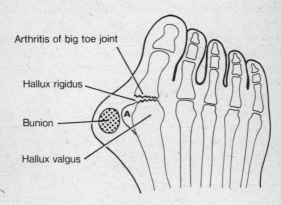

Fig. 28. The foot
Illustrating hallux valgus, hallux rigidus, arthritis of the big toe joint and a bunion.

Although hammer toe operations seldom cause disability lasting more than three to four weeks, operations to straighten the big toe and remove bunions take much longer and full recovery cannot be expected under three to four months.

Hallux valgus and bunions

This deformity can be corrected by removing the prominent lump of bone A (Fig. 28) and straightening the toe by removal of part of the first bone of the toe. This is either shortened or sometimes replaced by a small artificial spacer.

Hallux rigidus

A similar operation is used for the painful stiff rigid big toe joint. Part of the bone is removed and nowadays is frequently replaced by a plastic spacer which frees the joint but maintains reasonable length of the toe.

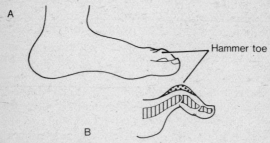

Fig. 29. Hammer toe
As shown in B, there is often a development of hardened skin on top.

Hammer toe

In this condition the bones of the toe which form the first toe joint are fixed in a bent position. The toe is straightened by removing the prominent parts of the bones which form this joint and temporarily fixing them together with a wire threaded along the bones. This stays in place till the joint is fixed.

HEEL PAIN

People suffering from generalised arthritis often complain of pain in the heel but it is often the result of simple over-use

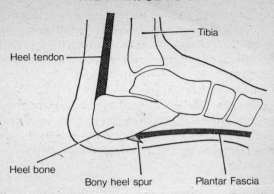

Fig. 30.   The foot and heel
Showing the bones, tendons, and the bony heel
spur which sometimes develops.

and the modern craze for jogging may be the start of
troublesome symptoms in an older person who is overweight
and overdoes it.

There are two distinct sites of pain in the heel.

1.   *Tendonitis*

At the attachment of the Achilles' tendon to the heel bone,
the tendon becomes swollen and tender and is painful when
stretched or the calf muscle contracts to pull up the heel.
Doctors call this condition tendonitis. Sometimes the bursa
or small sac of fluid which separates the tendon from the heel
bone becomes swollen and inflamed.

Rest, avoiding strenuous games and raising the heel of the
shoe to relax the inflamed tendon will probably be sufficient
in mild cases but in more intractable cases various types of
physiotherapy – of which ultrasound is probably the most
effective – should be tried. Hydrocortisone injections into the
tissues around the tendon often produce a dramatic cure.

The heel tendon is a common site to be affected by gout.
This condition often takes a long time to settle down.

2.   *Plantar fasciitis*

Here the pain is experienced under the heel where the long

plantar ligament, one of the main supporters of the arch of the foot, is attached to the heel bone. It may occur spontaneously in heavily built people who stand for long periods when it is due to a continued strain of the plantar ligament. In some cases the pull of the ligament on the bone produces a spur of bone projecting down from the heel bone and this in itself may be the cause of persistent pain.

In other cases it may be one of the earliest signs of rheumatoid arthritis, particularly if it affects both feet.

Treatment

Simple measures include the use of a soft sponge-rubber pad in the heel or, if there is evidence of flat foot, an insole should be used to support the long arch and exercises practised to strengthen the small muscles of the foot.

If the pain persists, injections of a mixture of hydro-cortisone and a local anaesthetic will often clear up the condition. Very occasionally, if the bony spur under the heel is the obvious cause of the pain, it may be necessary to operate on the heel and remove the projecting piece of bone.

Chiropody

Arthritis of the foot or toes often causes deformities of the joints with bony prominences which are constantly irritated by the pressure of shoes. These are frequently seen on the inner side of the big toe, the top of the other toes or underneath the fore-part of the foot. The overlying skin becomes thickened and harder producing a painful callosity and sometimes the skin breaks down to form an ulcer. These bony prominences and deformities cannot always be corrected and operations are certainly inadvisable in the presence of diabetes or a poor blood supply to the feet.

Considerable relief can, however, often be provided by wearing softer comfortable roomy shoes and appropriate pad-ding with soft wool or sponge rubber pads. This is a job for an expert chiropodist and anyone suffering from corns, callosities and troublesome toe-nails should certainly seek treatment from a chiropodist who in the U.K. may work privately or at one of the Hospital or Local Authority Foot Clinics.

11

THE PAINFUL SHOULDER

Pain in the shoulder is common and the cause is often obscure and difficult to localise. General disorders and diseases affecting nearby structures, e.g. the neck, the lungs or heart may first appear as pain in the shoulder. There are three separate joints around the shoulder, any of which may be the site of arthritic changes. In addition various tendons related to the joint may be the site of degeneration or inflammation. See Fig. 6 on page 19.

Causes of pain in the shoulder

1.   *Referred pain*
   Arthritis of the joints in the neck or injury and degenerative changes in the cartilage discs of the cervical spine can cause irritation of the nerves emerging from your neck with pain referred to your shoulder.

2.   *Arthritis* of the joints around your shoulder
   In addition to the shoulder joint between the upper end of your humerus and your shoulder blade, there are two other joints - one between your breast bone (or sternum) and your collar bone (clavicle) and another between part of your shoulder blade known as the acromion and the outer end of your collar bone. Any or all of these joints may be affected in generalised rheumatoid arthritis or may be the site of osteo-arthritis.

3.   *Degenerative changes* in the tendons and the capsule of your shoulder joint.
   The upper end of the humerus and the socket of your shoulder blade are held together by a strong fibrous capsule.

Passing over this capsule are two important tendons which are often involved in degenerative changes which cause you pain on particular movements of your shoulder.

(a)   The *supraspinatus tendon*, which passes from the muscles of the shoulder blade and is attached to the upper end of your humerus, is very liable to wear and tear with continued use of your shoulder, particularly in older people. You feel a sharp pain over the top of the shoulder when lifting the arm away from the side.

(b)   The *biceps tendon* which runs in a groove in front of and above your shoulder. This tendon may become thickened and tender and occasionally ruptures completely. In addition to the tenderness, pain is felt when lifting your arm forwards.

These tendons blend with the capsule of the joint and when they are injured or begin to degenerate they set up a chronic inflammation of the capsule of your shoulder. This is an example of non-articular rheumatism as opposed to true arthritic changes of your shoulder joint itself.

4.   *Frozen shoulder*

This is one of the commonest causes of a stiff painful shoulder.

The condition may follow an injury but often occurs spontaneously, particularly if, for one reason or another you are unable to move your shoulder fully, e.g. following a stroke, a chest operation or heart disease.

The main complaint is pain in your shoulder which is made worse by movement and in spite of all forms of treatment the condition may last for many months. Fortunately in most cases the condition gradually improves and movement slowly returns.

Treatment of the frozen shoulder

When your shoulder is painful and tender, your arm should be rested in a full sling, and you will need simple pain-killing tablets for the first two or three weeks.

As the pain settles gradually mobilising exercises and short-wave diathermy will help to restore movement to the joint. These should not be forced but some assistance will be required. Practise pendulum exercises while leaning forward to the affected side. Follow this by assisted exercises. From the horizontal position, lift your arm from the side and forwards and backwards, and attempt to touch the small of your back and the back of your neck. See Fig. 23, page 63.

Occasionally in very intractable cases when a particular movement cannot be achieved, a manipulation of the joint under an anaesthetic is helpful. This may be combined with an injection of a local anaesthetic and hydrocortisone into the joint.

Prevention

One of the most important things is to prevent the stiffness occurring and anyone suffering from an injury, a degree of paralysis or other illness which inhibits movement of the shoulder, should be helped and shown how to keep the shoulder as mobile as possible by supervised active and passive movements.

Shoulder-hand disorder

Sometimes a painful stiff shoulder is associated with pain referred down the arm into the hand which becomes swollen and blue from disease. Your fingers stiffen, the muscles waste and the skin is tender, giving rise to a fairly useless arm. You should be encouraged to exercise and use your hand by local heat and exercises. There is often a psychological disturbance which may require special treatment.

Arthritis of the shoulder

Any or all of the three joints involved in movement of the shoulder may be affected by either rheumatoid arthritis or osteo-arthritis.

Sterno-clavicular joint

This is the joint between the inner end of the collar bone or clavicle, and the breast bone or sternum, and is often one of the earliest joints to be involved in generalised rheumatoid arthritis. Swelling of this joint is easily visible and because the clavicle has to move whenever your arm is moved, pain is felt on vigorous movements of your arm.

The acromic-clavicular joint

The joint between the outer end of your collar bone and your shoulder blade is called the acromic-clavicular joint. This joint is often injured in strenuous games, and later in life arthritis of the joint may develop, causing thickening and pain above your shoulder on full movement of your arm.

The shoulder joint

This is the main joint at which movement of your arm takes place. It is formed by the rounded head of the upper end of the humerus fitting into the shallow socket at the upper and outer end of your shoulder blade.

Normally there is a wide range of movement of this joint in all directions. It is the commonest joint in the body to be dislocated and, because it is very liable to injury, osteo-arthritic changes may develop in later life with stiffness and pain on movement.

In common with other joints in the body where a wide range of movement occurs, your shoulder is often affected in rheumatoid arthritis. The joint becomes swollen and movements increasingly limited while the X-ray shows signs of destruction of the articular cartilage. In advanced cases your shoulder becomes extremely painful and your arm is held to the side of your body. The resulting stiffness prevents your hand reaching the top of your head or the small of your back.

Treatment of the arthritic shoulder

Various forms of physiotherapy, e.g. short-wave diathermy and progressive shoulder exercises, may help to restore some movement, and intra-articular hydrocortisone injections will help to reduce the swelling and relieve the pain.

Surgical treatment

If these measures fail and shoulder pain continues and it becomes increasingly difficult to use your arm then operative treatment must be considered.

Arthroplasty

Replacement of the joint by an artificial shoulder may

dramatically relieve pain but because of the difficulty of re-attaching the muscles to the metal head of the humerus, improvement in the range of movement is limited. There are also difficulties in fixing the prosthesis to the fragile bones of your shoulder and humerus and the long-term results are sometimes disappointing.

Osteotomy

In view of these technical difficulties of shoulder joint replacement the operation of osteotomy, dividing the bones above and below the joint, is sometimes performed. As in other joints it relieves the pain and this relief is often accompanied by an improved range of movement. Until the technical difficulties of joint replacement have been solved it is probably the best way of restoring some useful function to a shoulder joint which has been irretrievably damaged by arthritis.

Arthrodesis

When the joint is severely disorganised an arthrodesis or stiffening operation is sometimes used. This will relieve the pain completely and although all shoulder joint movement disappears the arm fixed to the shoulder blade is still capable of a useful range of movement because almost half the range of arm movement normally occurs between the shoulder blade and the chest wall.

12

PAIN IN THE ELBOW

Tennis elbow

Pain in your elbow may be due to osteo-arthritis which often follows an old injury or fracture involving the joint. It may also be affected in generalised rheumatoid arthritis when the joint becomes painful and swollen and movement is limited.

But the commonest cause of a painful elbow is the condition known as tennis elbow. As its name implies, it often affects people who play a lot of tennis but any continued unaccustomed prolonged use of the elbow, e.g. hedge-cutting with shears, may give rise to the typical symptoms.

You feel the pain at or just below the sharp bony prominence on the outer side of the joint, which is tender and occasionally swollen, and the pain radiates down the outer side of your forearm and is made worse if you contract the muscles on the back of your forearm as when playing a backhand shot in tennis. It is due to a strain or tear of the muscles of your forearm which are attached to this ridge of bone, or to some inflammation and thickening of the synovial lining on the outer side of the joint.

A similar condition occurs less frequently on the inner side of the elbow and this is called a Golfer's Elbow. Here the flexor muscles in front of your forearm are more likely to be involved, giving rise to pain and tenderness over the bony prominence on the inner side. The condition often settles down without any particular treatment if you give up sport or gardening for a while, and wear a firm elastic arm band below the elbow which often relieves the pain and allows reasonable use of the arm.

If the pain persists in spite of rest, an injection of a local anaesthetic and hydrocortisone into the painful area will often cure this troublesome condition. The injection sometimes causes a temporary worsening of the pain and it may require repeating two or three times.

A similar pain may be referred down the arm from the arthritic condition of the neck. It is associated with some neck stiffness, and intermittent traction or a manipulation of the neck will often give relief.

ARTHRITIS OF THE ELBOW

Osteo-arthritis

The elbow joint is frequently injured in childhood. Dislocation or fractures around the joint may cause some permanent irregularity resulting in osteo-arthritis of the elbow in later life. Over the years the joint becomes progressively stiffer and more painful, particularly in people who do heavy manual work.

Rheumatoid arthritis

The elbow joint may also be involved in rheumatoid arthritis. The joint becomes swollen and tender and movements limited and painful. The early symptoms usually settle with rest, avoiding vigorous movements and simple anti-rheumatic drugs, but occasionally operative treatment may be required. When the joint is very swollen a synovectomy operation, removing the thickened inflamed synovial membrane, may relieve the symptoms considerably.

If X-rays show that the joint surfaces have been badly destroyed, and movement is consistently painful, removal of a part or the whole of the joint may be indicated.

In the past a complete replacement operation of the elbow joint has not been particularly successful as the implant tends to loosen with use, but recent developments are proving more successful.

13

EMOTIONAL FACTORS IN ARTHRITIS

Anyone who has been involved in the care of a patient suffering from chronic arthritis either as a relative, a nurse or a doctor will be aware of the close connection between their emotional state and the severity of the symptoms. There is a physical explanation for this. Periods of anxiety, embarrassment and grief stimulate the endocrine glands which affect the secretion of hormones and the normal contraction of small blood vessels, and this in turn aggravates the pain in rheumatic joints.

You may be anxious because of an unhappy home life, or financial worry. It could be a feeling of helplessness that it is becoming impossible to cope with a house and family responsibilities, and the fear of becoming a helpless cripple. It is very important to be optimistic about the future, help *yourself*, and remain as active as possible. Relatives and friends should never encourage a sheltered existence and must help to preserve as much independence as possible.

The use of tranquillisers, e.g. Valium, and mild sedation at night may often help to tide you over these periods of depression but there is a very real danger of addiction to these drugs and they should never be used for prolonged periods.

Occasionally, generalised arthritis is associated with more serious forms of depression requiring the use of some of the more potent anti-depressive drugs, and then the physician in charge of the case may seek the help of a psychiatrist.

The degree to which mental disturbances aggravate rheumatism will vary from one person to another. Some people with a minor rheumatic disorder take to their bed and become virtually helpless, while others with severe crippling joint disease struggle on running a home and looking after the family.

Managing such cases calls for all the skill and ingenuity of an experienced physician and the whole-hearted support of other members of the family.

14

UNORTHODOX MEDICINE AND NEW DEVELOPMENTS

Natural food and herbs

Doctors in training are taught a system of medicine which is based on a long and careful study of the anatomy and function of all the organs of the human body. This is the basis of orthodox medicine as practised throughout most of the civilised world. Side by side with this system are others based on theories not held by most doctors but providing a wide range of treatment which have come to be known as "fringe medicine".

Nature cure

This term includes the use of so-called natural foods, i.e. food grown without the aid of fertilisers and unadulterated with preservatives and often eaten raw, and is often combined with exposure of the body to sunlight and fresh air.

For some this is a way of life but others take a "nature cure" for two or three weeks a year at some expensive clinic where a strict and simple diet combined with massage, baths and other forms of physiotherapy will help to reduce weight. This alone will help anyone suffering from rheumatism or arthritis, but it is essential to continue dieting if any lasting benefit is to be achieved.

Herbal medicine and folk lore

A vast range of herbal remedies has been used for centuries for the cure of every disease, dating back to Chinese remedies 4,000 years ago.

Many of these were brought back to Europe during the voyages of discovery in the 15th and 16th centuries, and in 1616 Nicholas Culpeper, a physician in the City of London, published his book "Herbal" which was the basis of treatment with herbal extracts for the next 300 years. One of the most popular remedies was the plant rhubarb which in the 18th century was used as a cure for almost all diseases.

Although the claims of herbal treatment were often grossly exaggerated commercially, many of them have provided the basis for the manufacture of modern drugs once the active ingredient of the plant has been isolated in the laboratory. The best known example of this is the common foxglove, a decoction of which was used for the treatment of heart failure, from which the essential element – digoxin – was extracted, providing us with one of our most effective drugs.

Rubbing the painful area with a variety of home-made liniments, usually those producing some irritation of the skin (such as mustard) is a traditional and often effective way of relieving local pain.

Among a host of popular remedies for arthritis are honey, which is also used for many disorders, and apple cider vinegar, the acid content of which is said to help digestion. There is no real evidence that either of these help rheumatic sufferers in any way.

Most of you will have met someone who swears by the copper bracelet which has protected them from rheumatism for years and they provide popular gifts, particularly if they have been brought from some remote part of the world. Unfortunately they are too often to be seen in the doctor's surgery worn by people consulting him for rheumatic aches and pains.

Spa treatment

"Taking the waters" either by drinking large quantities of hot mineral water or taking a dip in a hot pool is a very old traditional form of treatment for rheumatism. It was popular with the early Greeks and Romans and with the expansion of the Roman Empire elaborate centres of relaxation with pools were built all over Europe. One of the best preserved is at Bath, which in the 18th century was rebuilt with elegant crescents around the Pump Room. It became very fashionable, attracting the nobility who came to take the cure for all manner of diseases.

One of the most popular of these places was at Spa in Belgium, and several similar centres which sprang up in Britain, e.g. Buxton, Harrogate, Leamington and Droitwich, also became known as spas. They all had a natural source of pure water of high mineral content and which was often heated. The contents of these spring waters have been fully analysed and although there is no evidence that they have any specific medicinal effect they are one part of a course of treatment that undoubtedly benefits sufferers from chronic arthritis.

Hydrotherapy

The important part of treatment in a spa is bathing in a warm pool which partly supports the body weight and allows the damaged joints to move freely and the weakened muscles to be exercised and strengthened. When the water contains a high concentration of salt the body is completely buoyant and no effort is expended on keeping afloat. These brine baths can, however, be very irritant to the nose and eyes. Other variations of pool treatment include spraying the painful area with water under pressure and in Continental clinics local heat is often applied in the form of a mud or peat bath.

There is no doubt that the relaxed and pleasant atmosphere of a spa, the routine exercises and constant attention combined with a strict diet will often greatly improve sufferers from rheumatism both physically and psychologically. Unfortunately in Britain most of the spas are no longer supported by the N.H.S. and are closing down, whereas those on the Continent are still very popular.

New drugs

In assessing the safety and value of drugs, stringent trials, beginning with animal experiments, are carried out. Once their safety has been established and there is some evidence that they are likely to be effective, studies using human patients begin with their full consent. This consists of a "double blind trial", in which half the patients are given the active substance under trial and half a placebo – a harmless but ineffective preparation – and the results are carefully examined at the end of a fixed period by means of a range of tests which have been carefully worked out beforehand. Such experiments are sponsored and supported by the Arthritis and Rheumatism Council and various University and Medical Research teams and involve a great deal of work and experience in assessing the results. It is, however, essential that all so-called "cures" should be scientifically investigated if we are to make any progress in helping people suffering from the ravages of arthritis without doing them any harm.

One of the latest products which received considerable publicity is an extract from a shellfish grown in New Zealand waters known as the New Zealand green-lipped mussel. The mussels are cultivated on marine farms which have a constant flow of unpolluted sea water, and an uncontaminated freeze-dried powder rich in amino-acids and minerals is produced. This is called seatone. Its anti-arthritic properties were discovered during screening of different types of shellfish in a search for a possible treatment for cancer and leukaemia. It has been claimed that the majority of sufferers either from rheumatoid or osteo-arthritis obtain relief from pain and stiffness after taking the extract in tablet form for two or three weeks.

Research into its effectiveness and its mode of action is being carried out in laboratories throughout the world. This extract has recently been subjected to a controlled clinical trial conducted by the Department of Rheumatology, Barts Hospital, using seatone and an identical harmless but inactive capsule in 30 patients suffering from rheumatoid arthritis. There was no significant difference between the patients taking seatone and the placebo tablets as regards pain and stiffness of the affected joints. This suggests that it is one of the many substances which have appeared on a wave of publicity only to disappear in a few years.

BONE-SETTERS

Osteopaths and chiropractics
The human frame is a series of inter-connected links which

up to middle age move smoothly in response to contraction of the muscles. As a result of injury, arthritic changes or increasing age the smooth joint surfaces become irregular, the muscles weaken and the ligaments are less elastic. As a result joints tend to stiffen and become painful on certain movements and nowhere is this seen more commonly than in the spine which has a very large number of small joints.

When there is no underlying disease many of these symptoms can be relieved at least temporarily by a manipulation of the affected area. By manipulation we mean an attempt by a bone-setter or doctor trained in this technique to move one bone on another, often through a very small range of movement, either to restore a minor displacement or to increase the range of movement by stretching the capsule or ligaments of a joint which has become shortened or adheres to other structures.

For many years certain individuals have acquired wide reputations as people skilled in the art of manipulation. This facility often ran in families and two very famous orthopaedic surgeons, Sir Robert Jones and his uncle Hugh Owen Thomas, were both descended from a long line of bone-setters from North Wales. The medical profession has been slow to adopt these techniques but there are now many medical practitioners who practise manipulative treatment to relieve chronically painful backs and other joints.

There are so many different groups of people practising this type of treatment that the average person is very confused. Let us see if we can clarify the picture.

The bone-setters or manipulators

These are people without any medical qualification or special training who confine themselves to treating stiff and painful joints and sometimes fractures by manipulation. They became skilled in the art and were usually able to diagnose and select the right sort of case for treatment but occasionally manipulated a diseased or inflamed joint with disastrous results.

In spite of the undoubted success of such unqualified manipulators as Sir Herbert Barker, the medical profession failed to recognise them officially, although an increasing number of doctors studied the techniques and practised manipulative treatment alongside orthodox medicine.

Osteopathy

In the U.S.A. about 100 years ago Dr. Andrew Taylor Still became disillusioned with orthodox treatment when his three children died during an outbreak of spinal meningitis. His studies of the structure of the spinal cord led him to the conclusion that minor dislocations of the joints affected the normal flow of blood at that particular area and if this was restored by manipulation the body would be able to deal with any disease. He claimed that manipulative treatment which he called osteopathy would cure all sorts of conditions such as digestive disturbances, gall stones and many others not normally connected with the musculo-skeletal system.

Because of this unorthodox view osteopathy has not been officially recognised in this country, although it is fully recognised in America where Schools of Osteopathy exist side by side with orthodox schools of medicine.

Chiropractic

There is another school of manipulative treatment very popular in the U.S.A. known as chiropractic. The theory behind this type of practice is that the spinal manipulation by correcting minor displacements cures the disease, not by allowing better blood circulation, but by speeding up nerve impulses.

In spite of considerable medical opposition chiropractic is now fully recognised in every state of the Union and the practitioners also have the right to sign death certificates.

So where do you look for treatment among such confusion? Here are some simple hard and fast rules.

1.   Any persistent complaint should in the first place be fully investigated by a registered medical practitioner. In the U.K., the N.H.S. provides everyone with a General Practitioner who has ready access to the full range of hospital services and Consultants. It is no good having your spine manipulated if

you suffer from diabetes, heart disease, rheumatoid arthritis or cancer!

2.   Once organic disease has been excluded and the symptoms have not responded to medical treatment and are confined to the spine or joints, manipulation is one type of treatment to be considered.

3.   Many physiotherapists attached to hospitals or in private practice are trained and skilled in manipulation of the spine or other painful joints, and manipulation will often form part of their treatment together with various types of heat and traction to the joints.

4.   Such treatment is carried out under the supervision of specialists in physical medicine or orthopaedic surgeons, a number of whom specialise in manipulative techniques and who have formed a professional body – the British Osteopathic Association. These are the doctors who together with their trained staff provide the right sort of manipulative treatment when it is indicated.

5.   There are in addition a large number of non-medical manipulators, osteopaths and chiropractics practising in this country whose skill and training vary considerably. There is a British School of Osteopathy which has a general Council and maintains a Register of fully trained osteopaths.

There is no doubt that many people are relieved of their chronic aches and pains by manipulative treatment. Provided extravagant claims are avoided, attempts are not made to cure all manner of diseases, and more serious organic diseases have been eliminated, fully trained osteopaths will continue to provide an essential service.

In the U.K. there are not enough medical practitioners or physiotherapists with a full training in manipulative techniques to serve fifty million people, and the interest of the general public would best be served in many areas by greater collaboration between the trained osteopath and orthodox medicine.

15

THE OUTLOOK

Nowadays the press, radio and particularly television explain the latest advances in medical treatment and most people want to know from their doctor what they are suffering from and whether these new lines of treatment can help them.

Operations to replace worn out joints have a dramatic appeal but because Mrs. Jones down the road who had a painful limp for many years is now walking well after her operation it does not necessarily mean that your aching joint will respond in the same way.

Medicine is not an exact science and a purely mechanistic approach can be dangerous. First we have to try and find out why your joints or your back are aching – sometimes, even after full investigation, no cause can be found, and even when it is established there may be no effective cure available. Then we have to rely on treating the symptoms with pain-relieving drugs and physical means.

It is fortunate that in the broad field of rheumatic and arthritic conditions the majority of symptoms disappear spontaneously either temporarily or permanently and this applies particularly to back pain.

People with a persistent pain or a swollen joint worry about themselves and develop anxiety symptoms that they are developing rheumatoid arthritis and will become increasingly crippled. They nearly always have a relative who is severely disabled with arthritis.

If full investigation shows there is nothing to suggest rheumatoid disease it is very important that they be reassured as soon as possible and in many cases the symptoms will disappear. Reassurance is one of the most effective and universal remedies.

The body is not a simple machine but an infinitely involved and delicate mechanism, and when it goes wrong there are no certain cures. In arthritis we have not yet achieved a drug which will cure the disease and operations are basically a very crude attempt at restoring the beautifully constructed design of the human joint. Most treatments have some side-effects and when a physician offers drug treatment, or a surgeon an operation, they both hope that the benefits will be considerable and the complications or side-effects few. But no treatment is without some side-effects, even the simple aspirin.

The spectrum of the rheumatic and arthritic diseases is very wide and there is no simple treatment that stands pre-eminent. In no other condition is the art of medicine displayed so clearly. In most cases there is a choice of treatments which work in different ways and which have to be altered according to the response of the individual and the stage of the disease. That is why in intractable cases of rheumatoid arthritis it is important that your treatment remains under the guidance of a rheumatologist who from his extensive past experience can decide that treatment *A* is more likely to help than treatment *B*. The various drugs used in the treatment of rheumatoid arthritis all have side-effects which vary in intensity from one person to another. This is why it is so important to maintain continuity of treatment either from your own G.P. or the doctor in charge of the Hospital Rheumatology Clinic so that you can quickly report any troublesome effects of the drug.

Surgery

We have already discussed some of the operations used to relieve the pain and disability from advanced arthritis of joints. Many of the operations used in the treatment of arthritic conditions are of a relatively minor character. They are rarely followed by any complications and the relief they afford is usually effective and quick. Among these are the tendon release operations for a trigger finger or thumb, division of the carpal ligament at the wrist for compression of the median nerve and synovectomies and reconstruction of stretched ligaments for arthritic changes in the hand.

This last operation is sometimes used just to improve the appearance of your hand. If, however, you can use the hand quite well it is doubtful whether surgical correction of the deformity is justified as some loss of function occasionally results.

Operations on the foot for arthritic deformities with painful areas should not be embarked on lightly by older people. Make every effort to relieve the discomfort by padding the toes, sponge rubber insoles and special shoes with soft uppers and a cellular rubber support in the heel and sole to act as shock absorbers.

Even in younger people the rate of recovery from toe and foot operations is often a good deal slower than anticipated and it may well be three or four months before you get back to full work.

Operations on the main weight-bearing joints – the hip and the knee – are major procedures and must always be preceded by a full medical check-up.

Diseases of the musculo-skeletal system are seldom fatal and these are not life-saving procedures when compared with those on the heart, lungs and kidneys. Operations designed to relieve pain and increase the range of movement can greatly improve the quality of life but they carry small but significant risks and before you embark on these big operations you must be convinced that your incapacity to get about or the continued pain are making life intolerable.

The results of total hip replacement, which is by far the commonest operation for the painful arthritic hip joint, are excellent but even this operation is occasionally complicated by loosening of the joint components or infection of the wound. Like all major operations on the pelvis or lower limb, it carries a slight risk of the patient developing a pulmonary embolus or clot on the lung which may be fatal.

These are all rare complications; the complication rate varies from approximately 2% to 10%, and they are more likely to occur in the elderly bed-ridden person.

These complications have the additional disadvantage that, if things do go wrong, repeat operations to restore the joint are difficult and more hazardous than the first operation.

Of the various operations to replace arthritic joints with artificial joints, that for the hip joint is by far the most successful. Anyone over the age of 50 with a diseased hip giving rise to increasing pain and disability, provided their general health is good, can undergo an operation to replace the joint with every confidence of being able to lead a reasonably active life provided they do not subject it to continued stresses and strains. They should particularly avoid jumping from a height.

Because these artificial joints may give rise to some trouble ten to fifteen years later, the operation is less frequently performed in younger people when some less extensive procedure may be used to tide them over until they are older.

Once you have decided to have an operation there are certain things you can do to help your recovery.*

Before operation
a)   Avoid chest infections and give up smoking.
b)   Operations are much more difficult in fat people so reduce your weight as much as possible.
c)   Learn to sleep on your back with the affected leg resting on a pillow.
d)   You will need a high comfortable chair and a fairly high bed with a foam mattress so you can slide out of bed and stand up more easily.
e)   A rubber bathmat will give you greater confidence when getting in and out of the bath but a shower is better than a bath for the first three months.
f)   Handles fixed to the wall in the loo will enable you to get on and off the lavatory as hip movements will be limited for a few months.
g)   Septic teeth should be dealt with well before the date of your operation.

---

* I am indebted to Mr. R. Denham, Consultant Orthopaedic Surgeon, Portsmouth for permission to take extracts from his booklet "How To Be A Successful Hippie" (Operative Treatment For The Painful Hip By Total Joint Replacement), which he gives to patients undergoing replacement surgery of the hip.

At the pre-operative assessment clinic

Report any septic spots, abrasions or sore toes. Let the doctor know about any unusual symptoms. e.g. fainting attacks, asthma, sensitivity to iodine or any particular drugs. You must also tell him about any drugs you are taking and particularly whether you are or have been taking cortisone or other powerful anti-rheumatic drugs.

After operation

An operation to replace the hip joint is a big operation and the tissues around the joint must be allowed to heal well before anything like a full range of movement is attempted. It will take at least six months before normal use of the joint is reached and elbow crutches should be used for the first month followed by two sticks for another month and then one stick in the opposite hand to the operated side for up to six months.

Subsequent progress

The most striking effect is the early disappearance of the aching discomfort and sharp jabs of pain on movement. The limp has become a habit and will disappear more slowly but most people will be able to walk almost normally in six months depending on how severe the deformity was before the operation.

You will have expert help with supervised exercises before and after the operation but treatment is not usually required after leaving hospital. Regular morning and afternoon walks on level ground, swimming and gentle golf should complete your rehabilitation and you should have a good serviceable hip joint for at least ten years. Take it all slowly and gradually.

The knee joint

The results of total replacement of the arthritic knee joint are by no means as successful as that for the hip. In spite of a great deal of research and a wide variety of artificial joints, problems have arisen, partly because the joint is more complex than the hip and also because it lies so near the surface of the skin. Nevertheless many good results have been achieved and research continues.

At the moment its use is largely confined to provide a useful range of movement in the very disorganised lax knee joint which often occurs in both knees in advanced rheumatoid arthritis. For the younger patient with an osteo-arthritic joint either an osteotomy below the knee or a double osteotomy above and below the knee is frequently used to re-align any deformity and relieve pain in the knee.

Total replacement of some other arthritic joint, e.g. the ankle joint, the elbow joint and shoulder joint is performed occasionally. These joints are often affected in advanced rheumatoid arthritis and the mechanical problems of fixing the small artificial joints to the bone are gradually being solved and an increasing number of these joints are being inserted.

The other joints affected in generalised rheumatoid arthritis are the small joints of the fingers and wrist. These joints are frequently destroyed in advanced arthritis resulting in considerable deformity. They can be successfully replaced by a plastic mobile spacer which re-aligns the bone and restores a useful range of painless movement.

As a result of widespread publicity in the press and television there is a general impression that replacing worn out joints is a simple mechanical problem with remarkably successful results.

However, the bonding of living tissue to metallic and plastic material has not been completely solved and gives rise to complications from time to time.

The replacement of several arthritic joints is a major undertaking and you should never attempt to over-persuade a surgeon to operate against his better judgement. An experienced surgeon often finds that he has to reduce a patient's expectations of surgery and may refuse to operate unless convinced that the pain and disability are severe and permanent.

Remember that the vast majority of aches and pains which we call rheumatism or arthritis clear up completely with simple measures: a period of rest for swollen and acutely painful joints with analgesics followed by graduated exercises and use.

In only a small proportion of cases do the symptoms persist

and the joints remain swollen. This is the time to consult your G.P. If the symptoms do not settle fairly soon further investigations will be required at the Rheumatology Clinic of your nearest hospital.

Do not despair - this is not a life or death disease and modern treatment is on the whole very effective.

We must maintain a spirit of optimism. A great deal of research is going on throughout the world and I am sure a cure for rheumatoid arthritis is not far away. Surgery for this disease is on the whole a helpful but temporary stage in the long journey to eradicate one of the oldest diseases.

APPENDIX I

Research into the causes of arthritis

Research in the United Kingdom is co-ordinated and financed by the Arthritis and Rheumatism Council whose funds are contributed almost entirely from voluntary sources. It is a measure of the widespread support that over 700 branches of the Council throughout the country raise over £700,000 per annum to finance research programmes and endow Professorial Chairs of Rheumatology in our Universities and Medical Schools. Much of this work is of a highly technical nature involving elaborate scientific techniques.

The various types of body cells concerned with the defence mechanism of the body when attacked by inflammation and their altered response to the new drugs used in treatment of rheumatic diseases are being closely examined. It has long been suspected that certain infective organisms or viruses play a part in the onset of rheumatoid arthritis and this possibility is being investigated at centres specially equipped for virological study.

Other centres are following up the discovery of an association between certain types of arthritis and inherited abnormalities of the blood groups to see if a genetic factor or heredity can explain the reason why some people develop the disease and others do not.

The structures which are so rapidly damaged and destroyed in rheumatoid arthritis are the cartilage and synovial membrane lining the joints. These changes are being studied by using the electron microscope and biochemical investigation at several important centres throughout the U.K.

These are a few examples of research into the cause of the disease but a great deal of work is going on into the treatment of the rheumatic diseases in collaboration with the pharmaceutical industry. The large drug companies, many of them multi-national, spend a great deal of money on developing and testing new drugs and making existing ones safer to use. They are often criticised because they make a substantial profit on the sale of some of their successful effective and often life-saving drugs, and because their work involves animal experiments. A large proportion of this profit is poured back into continued research and for every successful drug which is discovered there are literally hundreds which have to be discarded after a great deal of work has been done on their development and painstaking thorough testing. The use of small animals for studying the effect of drugs is absolutely essential if we are to make any progress in developing safe and effective drugs to relieve the pain and suffering and possibly cure the thousands of victims of this potentially crippling disease.

When cortisone was first introduced it proved to be the most powerful anti-inflammatory drug and its initial effect on a swollen painful joint was almost magical, but it proved to have very troublesome complications. Continued research by the drug firms has provided much safer drugs with a similar effect which can, under careful medical supervision, be given in small doses for long periods, and almost every month new anti-inflammatory drugs are put on the market which enable the rheumatologists to ring the changes and find the most suitable drug for individual patients.

Apart from supporting basic research projects into the cause of the disease and the development of effective drugs, the Council also supports the new Bio-engineering Departments which have brought together engineers and surgeons to study ways of reducing pressure on painful joints, or actually replacing the worn out human joint by an artificial joint made of plastic or metal material, or both. In other centres studies are going on to replace the diseased cartilage surface of affected joints by transplants of healthy cartilage.

Another very active field of research is that of suitable splints and other aids to living which restrict painful movements and thus enable patients to lead more active lives.

New plastic materials to provide light splints for such joints as the knee, ankle and wrist have been developed incorporating unobtrusive springs which permit controlled movement of disorganised joints.

The various types of physiotherapy are being studied to try and assess which are effective in relieving pain and increasing joint movement, and, in particular, strengthening the muscles controlling movement which rapidly waste when the joints are diseased.

These are but a few of the many research projects sponsored and supported by the Arthritis and Rheumatism Council, one of our most effective research organisations which thoroughly deserves full public support.

APPENDIX II

List of some of the Societies and Associations which provide help and information about rheumatism and arthritis.

ARTHRITIS AND RHEUMATISM COUNCIL, 8-10 Charing Cross Road, London, WC2H 0HN

The Council publishes useful booklets on various aspects of rheumatism and arthritis which are available free of charge and are designed to supplement advice given by your doctor. It also provides up-to-date information for General Practitioners and supports research projects into arthritic and rheumatic diseases. It sponsors many teaching programmes for doctors, medical students, nurses and physiotherapists and produces a series of valuable tape/slide programmes.

It is a charitable organisation depending on voluntary contributions and fully deserves every support. All donations and legacies are gratefully received.

BRITISH COUNCIL FOR REHABILITATION OF THE DISABLED, Tavistock House (South), Tavistock Square, London, WC1

This organisation is concerned with providing education and advice for all types of disabled people.

ARTHRITIS CARE, 1 Devonshire Place, London, W1N 2BD

Membership is open to anyone either suffering from or concerned with the problems associated with arthritis. They have about 100 centres which arrange outings and holidays at special hotels and organise social evenings.

THE BRITISH RED CROSS SOCIETY, 9 Grosvenor Crescent, London, SW1X 7EJ

This Society publishes a useful catalogue and supplies many different aids to help the disabled.

DISABLED LIVING FOUNDATION, 346 Kensington High Street, London, W14 8NS

The Foundation supplies up-to-date bulletins and booklets and has a permanent display of a full range of aids for disabled people.

THE DISABLEMENT RESETTLEMENT OFFICERS (D.R.O.s) at the Employment Exchanges arrange training in industrial rehabilitation units and help to settle disabled people in suitable employment. They can also arrange admission to various residential training centres, e.g.:

THE QUEEN ELIZABETH TRAINING COLLEGE FOR THE DISABLED, Leatherhead, Surrey, ST. LOYE'S COLLEGE FOR THE TRAINING AND REHABILITATION OF THE DISABLED, Exeter, and THE PORTLAND TRAINING COLLEGE FOR THE DISABLED, Harlow Wood, Mansfield, Nottinghamshire.

DRIVING FOR THE DISABLED:

The ability to drive a car makes all the difference between a confined sheltered existence and freedom and independence. There are a wide variety of alterations which can be applied to an ordinary car to enable a disabled person to drive and specially adapted invalid cars are also available. Two organisations provide services and advice:—

THE DISABLED DRIVERS ASSOCIATION, 4 Laburnum Avenue, Wickford, Essex

THE DISABLED DRIVERS MOTOR CLUB LTD., 39 Templewood, Ealing, London, W13 8BU

APPENDIX III

AIDS TO LIVING
Daily living can be made a good deal easier by a variety of aids and adaptations, many of which are available through the Local Authority. Most District General Hospitals have on their staff occupational therapists who will give advice about implements and appliances which will help you to lead an independent life.

AIDS TO WALKING
Walking sticks and elbow crutches:
These should be the correct height. When standing upright the tip should touch the ground with the elbow slightly bent and should be tipped with a rubber ferrule and have a padded handle. For frail elderly people a light quadruped walking stick (that is one with four feet) will give more stability and a better sense of security. A stick adapted with a pincer grip at the end will enable you to pick things up from the floor.
Walking frames:
These again must be the correct height and as light as possible consistent with strength and rigidity. Wheels should be avoided but arm rests in front will help the very disabled. This is known as a pulpit frame. Excellent light rigid aluminium sticks and frames which are completely adjustable are made by OEC Orthopaedic Ltd. and the frame is generally known as the Zimmer Frame.
Wheel-chairs:
These should always be self-propelled and should fold up. They are intended to help a patient to be wheeled out of doors and only in exceptionally severe cases should they be used indoors. You must retain your independence and ability to walk as much as possible.

ALTERATIONS TO THE HOME:
There are many problems and hazards in the home for the disabled, e.g. slippery floors, steep stairs, unguarded fires, poor lighting and electric plugs at floor level – these and many other difficulties may require attention.

Food preparation:

Lifting heavy pans with a rheumatic hand or fingers proves difficult. Pans should be as light as possible with big broad handles and you should learn to use the lever principle when raising the pan by resting the handle on the opposite forearm or wrist.

In fact all small handles should be avoided. Devices to thicken the shaft of a variety of implements including pens are available.

Spring clamps with handles for removing jar tops, a bread knife with a specially designed handle which can be slotted through a support containing the bread and a large wooden slot which can be put over a door key are two other examples of useful aids.

Aids to dressing:

High beds are much easier to manage than low ones. You should wear light warm clothing which is easily put on and taken off, and long-handled shoe-horns and a device with a handle and adjustable grip at the end will help to pull up socks, stockings and other garments.

Toilet facilities:

One of the most difficult housing problems is arranging a lavatory which is easily accessible. The seat may also require raising and both the bath and the toilet will usually require hand-rails.

Shoes:

Well-fitting comfortable shoes are essential and if necessary these should be ordered specially. Simple comfortable house-shoes can be rapidly moulded in Plastizote and if you have rheumatic deformities of the feet you should wear soft cellular soles and heels which act as shock absorbers. In addition to relieving pain in the feet they also help to protect arthritic knees and hips.

INDEX